WOMEN, DISABILITY AND MENTAL DISTRESS

Women, Disability and Mental Distress

Julia L.T. Smith

ASHGATE

Published by
Ashgate Publishing Limited
Wey Court East
Union Road
Farnham
Surrey, GU9 7PT
England

Ashgate Publishing Company
110 Cherry Street
Suite 3-1
Burlington, VT 05401-3818
USA

www.ashgate.com

British Library Cataloguing in Publication Data
A catalogue record for this book is available from the British Library

The Library of Congress has cataloged the printed edition as follows:
Smith, Julia L. T.
Women, disability and mental distress / by Julia L.T. Smith.
pages cm
Includes bibliographical references and index.
ISBN 978-1-4094-5400-7 (hardback) – ISBN 978-1-4094-5401-4 (ebook) – ISBN 978-1-4724-0709-2 (epub)
1. People with disabilities–Mental health–Great Britain. 2. Women with disabilities–Mental health–Great Britain. 3. People with disabilities–Mental health services–Great Britain. 4. Women with disabilities–Mental health services–Great Britain. I. Title.
RC451.4.H35S65 2015
362.2–dc23

2014028905

ISBN 9781409454007 (hbk)
ISBN 9781409454014 (ebk – PDF)
ISBN 9781472407092 (ebk – ePUB)

MIX
Paper from responsible sources
FSC® C013985
www.fsc.org

Printed in the United Kingdom by Henry Ling Limited,
at the Dorset Press, Dorchester, DT1 1HD

Contents

Acknowledgements

To each of the women who gave of their time to talk openly about their personal experiences of mental distress, a sincere debt of gratitude is owed as without their participation this book would not have been possible. In sharing their experiences, these women spoke of a hope that the book would serve to be a helpful and informative resource to professionals within mental health and social care who within their various roles sought to support disabled women who experience mental distress. Similarly, it was hoped that the book would be of help to disabled women who like themselves had experienced, or were experiencing mental distress and I hope on their behalf that these wishes will in the months and years ahead be achieved.

Secondly, to friends too numerous to mention who, throughout the writing process offered continuing encouragement and support and in so doing helped me to reach the finishing line a big thankyou to you all.

Finally, to close family and dear friends who, for over thirty years have unfailingly provided care, support, love and friendship this book is dedicated to you.

Introduction

Through the latter decades of the twentieth century within the UK, increasing amounts of attention began to be paid to meeting the individual support needs of both mental health service users and people with a physical impairment. Evidence of this can be found both in the expanding body of literature that had begun to examine mental health and physical impairment from a range of perspectives and the increased range of service provision offered by a growing number of health and social care providers for individuals within each group. In contrast, the mental and psychological health needs of individuals living with a physical impairment *and* who experience diagnosed mental distress have largely been overlooked by health and social care service providers, practitioners and organisations for whom the main focus or area of interest is either mental health or physical impairment. The lack of attention which historically has been paid, both in theory and in practice, to meeting the mental health needs of people with physical impairments who experience mental distress has resulted in the absence of a comprehensive knowledge base of how best to support such individuals which in turn has led to their mental health needs remaining neglected, and subsequently left unmet.

Likewise, the subject area of physical impairment and mental health had until the latter decades of the twentieth century received little attention within the academic, policy and research literatures but where it was examined, a medical approach was overwhelmingly adopted by the literature with physical impairments and mental health issues viewed as 'illnesses' or 'conditions' and with minimal focus on the individual per se. Predominantly, the literature has been underpinned by two key assumptions: firstly, that a physical impairment per se will be a cause of psychological distress and that affected individuals will need to adjust to their 'loss' in stages before they can become 'psychologically whole' again (Turner and Noh 1988); and secondly, that the solutions to an individual's mental distress are to be found within the individual and the text will examine both assumptions. In addition it will discuss literature which, in the latter decades of the twentieth century, in contrast to an entrenched medical perspective, began to examine the topic area of physical impairment and mental health from a *social* perspective. Within this literature attention began to be given to the potential for social and cultural barriers such as societal attitudes towards impairment or barriers to service provision to impact on the mental well-being of people living with physical impairments. In shifting the focus from an individual's *impairment* onto *disability*, the social model of disability (and its history and relevance within the context of women's personal experiences which will be discussed) uses the term to refer to disabling social, environmental and attitudinal barriers rather than a lack of functional ability.

The origins of my interest within the subject area of physical impairment and mental health are long held and primarily two-fold. Firstly, as a young teenager diagnosed with a spinal lesion that rapidly resulted in extensive functional paralysis, significant life changes and adjustments at both a physical and psychological level had to be made. A four year hospital admission following the onset of paralysis was punctuated by periods of both 'feeling low' and prolonged episodes of diagnosed clinical depression, but overwhelmingly any mental health or psychological needs were sidelined by medical professionals for whom the priority was the physical body and a desire to make it as 'well' and as 'normal' as possible. Thus, it was not until reaching adulthood that I was finally able to access mental health provisions which very belatedly enabled me to share thoughts, feelings and emotions about my grief and changed life circumstances.

Proceeding some years later to qualify as a social worker, my dual experiences of living with a physical impairment and experiencing mental distress proved to be invaluable in my work within an adult's physical disabilities team, working predominantly with women service users who either self-presented to seek mental health (and other) support or, having been referred by other health or social care agencies, were assessed as having mental health/psychological needs. A persistent lack of appropriate mental health provision for this group of women, combined with clear evidence of a stark delineation between physical disability services and mental health services across both the statutory and non-statutory sector was experienced both by myself, as a social care professional, and service users as being immensely frustrating and disappointing, and subsequently for large numbers of women resulted in their mental health needs being left unmet.

In addition to my involvement at both a personal and professional level with physical disability and mental health service providers over two decades, the origin of this text is founded upon a recent research study (Smith 2010) which examined the experiences of a group of women with physical impairments who had experienced mental distress. As users of mental health services, the research sought to determine from the women's personal viewpoints, whether mental health and allied professionals and the services and organisations in which they worked, had been effective in meeting their mental health needs. Additionally, the study endeavoured to identify whether women with congenital impairments and women with acquired impairments differed in their personal analysis of the relationship between physical impairment and mental distress whilst also examining whether they perceived social disability, for example, the attitudes of a majority able-bodied society towards physical impairment, to be a source of mental distress. Further, the study examined whether women with a range of physical impairments who had experienced mental distress, identified a shared set of barriers to accessing mental health service provision and finally, sought to determine whether mental health services in the years ahead could meet their mental health needs more appropriately, and if so, how?

In undertaking the study, a unique approach was utilised through incorporating both the experiences of physical impairment and mental distress of 12 women aged between 18 and 64, each living with a diagnosed permanent physical impairment. Additionally, each woman had previously been diagnosed on one or more occasions with a mental health condition for which treatment of some form had been received (and which for two women was ongoing). Women who had acquired a physical impairment as a consequence of mental distress, for example, paralysis resulting from a suicide attempt or, women with a history of mental distress prior to acquiring their impairment were not included within the selection criteria. All women were of British white ethnic origin, with six women born with their impairments and six living with acquired impairments. In seeking to recruit a sample group which reflected a spectrum of physical impairments and mental health conditions, neither the nature of the impairment or mental health condition was specified and subsequently included women living with spinal cord injuries, spina bifida and a spinal tumour whilst experiences of mental distress included acute clinical depression, self-harm, stress and anxiety and an eating disorder. Women who were mothers or had other care responsibilities and women who were single or had no dependents were all represented within the group.

In conducting the fieldwork stage of the study a mixed methods approach was used: face-to-face semi-structured interviews were conducted over a four-month period (with a minimum of two interviews per person), with a focus group having been held one month after completion of all interviews, its purpose being to explore issues that been generated through the interviews at a more strategic level (Hollis et al. 2002). In wishing to explore any regional variations in mental health provision, endeavours were made to recruit participants from across the UK whilst simultaneously balancing the time constraints for conducting fieldwork and practical travelling considerations for myself as a wheelchair-user researcher. Consequently, all participants lived within a 100-mile radius of Birmingham where the study was based.

In authoring a text which I consider to be both needed and long overdue, the book is seeking to be innovative in providing an in-depth discussion of a to date largely neglected area of personal experiences and in doing so it will hopefully additionally ignite discussion and meaningful debate about the subject area of women, disability and mental distress. In focusing on the subject area of physical impairment and mental distress, it is hoped the text will make an original and welcomed contribution to knowledge in relation to both policy and practice whilst simultaneously aiming to be of benefit and interest to a wide spectrum of health and social care professionals working within the fields of physical disability and/or mental health. Additionally, I hope it will become a valued text for both academics within the specialisms of counselling, social work, psychology, medicine, nursing, disability studies or mental health and to undergraduate and postgraduate students across these realms. Furthermore, placing the emphasis on a service user perspective will, I hope, position the text as an informative and helpful resource for women with physical impairments who seek support for mental distress. Whilst the text focuses predominantly on the personal experiences of disabled women, there exist many overlaps between women's experiences of working with mental health and allied professionals and the experiences of disabled men, and therefore it is hoped that the book will have worth for men with physical impairments also. Finally, whilst based on the findings of a UK study, I believe that much of the book's content will have relevance for other Western countries.

Chapter 1 will begin with an examination of a historical and widely held assumption within medical and psychology literatures that have examined the topic area of physical impairment and mental health, that individuals living with a physical impairment will inevitably experience mental distress (on one or more occasions) by virtue of living with an impairment. By providing evidence from the research undertaken, the chapter will highlight the problematic nature of the assumption of a causal link between living with a physical impairment and experiencing mental distress (overwhelmingly assumed to be depression). Secondly, the study's findings relating to the perceived potential of factors such as society's attitudes towards physical impairment, or the representation of disability within the media to impact on women's mental well-being and self-image will be discussed before finally examining the diverse ways in which women experienced their relationships with significant people in their lives within the context of their personal experiences of mental distress.

Within the limited literature to date which in recent decades has examined the topic area of accessing and using mental health services for disabled people, consistently it has highlighted the barriers that individuals had encountered and that the overall process of gaining access had been fraught with difficulties. Furthermore, where mental health services had been accessed, individuals had considered any provision to have been inappropriate for their needs (McKenzie 1992, Begum 1999, Morris 2004). Based on the study findings, Chapter 2 will therefore offer a detailed examination of women's experiences of both gaining access to and using mental health services across the statutory and non-statutory sectors. In particular, it will highlight how factors such as lengthy waiting times for initial assessments, difficult to access service information and a lack of psychological support within hospital rehabilitation units had affected women's ability to access service provision. Likewise the chapter will show how the professional's level of understanding and awareness of disability and impairment, and the length of contact time offered to an individual by a service or mental health professional, were clearly linked to women's rating of their experiences of using mental health services and their effectiveness in addressing their mental distress.

Over recent decades within the UK, the use of counselling as a form of treatment or psychological support has expanded significantly alongside the emergence of a growing body of literature which has examined the processes of counselling when working with diverse client groups or circumstances. Within the sample group, the majority of women had received counselling as part of their treatment for their mental distress but in comparison with other client groups, the body of counselling literature that focuses on working with people with physical impairments has historically been, and remains small. In Chapter 3, the counselling approaches that counsellors, psychologists and allied professionals have typically used when working with disabled clients will be examined, whilst the key criticisms, which over recent years have been directed at counselling responses to disability which predominantly have been founded upon loss theories such as their disempowering nature and their role in reinforcing the medical model of disability, will be discussed. In responding to the criticisms levelled at established theories of loss, recent years have witnessed the emergence of alternative approaches to loss, each of which have been presented as offering a more accurate and realistic explanation of how individuals respond to physical impairment and the merits of two key alternative approaches will be outlined. The concept of loss will then be considered from the viewpoints of the study participants.

Historically, the lack of counselling approaches which are informed by the social model of disability and which recognise the potential for oppression within the counsellor–client relationship has been widely claimed to have led to the long held stereotypes and prejudices around physical disability being left unchallenged. The final part of the chapter will thus consider counselling approaches which, in recent years, based on their core principles, have been advocated for use when working with disabled clients in addition to considering the potential benefits or otherwise of a disability counselling approach.

Further evidenced by the study data was the strong preference expressed by the large majority of women to work in counselling with a same gender counsellor and, within the context of the counselling process both being viewed positively and as having beneficial outcomes, a same gender counsellor was considered to be of significant importance. Chapter 4 will therefore firstly discuss the issue of gender, highlighting from the women's perspective the considered advantages and disadvantages of counsellors being the same gender as their clients. Secondly, the recently emerged and continuing debate (initially amongst disabled academics primarily, but more recently with welcome contributions from disabled people themselves (for example, Smith 2003, Reeve 2004, Jack 2009)) as to whether people with physical impairments are best served by working with counsellors who themselves have a physical impairment (or have either lived experience or a good understanding of physical impairment), as opposed to an able-bodied counsellor with no lived experience of impairment will be discussed. However, several women drew attention to the need to consider factors and attributes beyond gender and impairment which were believed to be equally important within the context of women's experiences of the counselling process such as the counsellors personality or character traits and their ability to listen to and communicate with their client and each of these factors will be considered. Finally, whilst Chapter 1 considered the impact (or potential impact) of factors such as societal attitudes towards impairment or the representation of disability in the media to affect women's mental well-being, Chapter 4 will finally examine women's recollections of their experiences of distress and the personal circumstances relevant to those experiences.

Evidenced consistently both within the research study's findings and within the limited available literature was how any positive experiences of working with counsellors or other mental health professionals had been closely linked to other factors such as a good working relationships between professional and client, the professional's level of understanding and awareness of disability and impairment related issues and their willingness to both listen to and value the disabled client's perspectives concerning their mental distress. Within Chapter 5 the focus will be an examination of mental health provisions in the years and decades ahead for women (and men) with physical impairments requiring mental health support, considering in detail a range of changes to the professional training courses of mental health and health and social care professionals who work, or may potentially work, with disabled clients. The importance of factors such as the inclusion of teaching both around the social model of disability and disability equality training within professional training courses, both within the context of the support provided by mental health professionals and the approaches used when working with people with physical impairments of either gender will also be discussed. Based on the study findings, the need for mental health professionals to have a greater awareness of the problematic representation of disability in the media and its potential to impact on mental well-being, alongside an awareness of the positive ways in which recent changes in disability legislation may have impacted on the mental well- being of disabled people was a widely shared view and both topics will be discussed.

In reaffirming that disabled people have historically encountered both in gaining access to and using mental health services over several decades, the final part of the chapter will discuss both the structural and organisational changes which women widely believed needed to take place in endeavouring to improve disabled people's experiences of accessing and using services and additionally to observe higher incidences of positive reported experiences of receiving appropriate mental health support which had been effective in addressing an individual's mental distress.

In bringing together the key themes and findings which emerged from the topic areas discussed within and across the individual chapters, the final chapter will consider the potential outcomes for mental health and allied professionals working within statutory and non-statutory sector organisations and services, and for the women (and men) with physical impairments with whom they work, if the changes which were identified as needing to take place, became reality. It will discuss how an increased awareness of the intersections between physical impairment and mental health could potentially result in the years ahead in significant positive and welcome changes to both service provision and service delivery and hopefully could steadily impact positively on the lives and mental well-being of women with physical impairments who experience mental distress.

Finally, before proceeding, a few words of explanation in relation to the language and terminology used within the book may help any readers who may question the use of some terminology which is used interchangeably throughout the text. Firstly, across the group there existed a broadly shared agreement of how *disability* and *impairment* were defined and therefore, for the purposes of this book, 'disability' will be defined as:

> The functional limitations within the individual caused by physical, mental or sensory impairment.
>
> Oliver 1996

Whilst the term 'impairment' will be defined as:

> The functional limitation within the individual caused by physical, mental or sensory impairment.
>
> Oliver 1996

Physical and social barriers are referred to as:

> Those that prevent the full participative citizenship of disabled people that marginalise and segregate people in every aspect of social life and that deny access to and participation in organisations and that preclude equal rights.
>
> Swain, French et al. 2004

The terms 'people/women with physical impairments' and 'disabled people/women' are used interchangeably as, whilst some women described themselves as 'a woman living with a physical impairment', others referred to themselves as 'a disabled woman'. Likewise, within the focus group, some women expressed a preference for the term 'a group of women with physical impairments', whilst others felt that, gathered together, they were 'a group of disabled women' so efforts have been made to accommodate the preferences of all research participants.

Chapter 1
Living with a Physical Impairment: Is Mental Distress Inevitable?

Introduction

Within this chapter the focus will be on three related areas. Firstly, it will discuss assumptions which, within some areas of the psychology and medical bodies of literature, have long been held relating to the inevitability of women (and men) who are living with physical impairments experiencing mental distress. Predominantly founded upon an assumption of a causal link between living with a physical impairment and experiencing mental distress, the problematic nature of an assumed causal link will be discussed, providing evidence from both my research and empirical studies which within recent decades have rejected a causal link between a lived experience of physical impairment and experiencing mental distress. Secondly, the chapter will discuss findings from the research with regard to the perceived potential of factors such as societal attitudes towards physical impairment and the broad representation of disability within the media and its potential to affect the mental well-being and self-image of disabled women in the early twenty-first century. Finally, the diverse ways in which individual women experienced their relationships with significant persons in their lives within the context of their experiences of mental distress will be examined.

Women with Physical Impairments and Mental Health

Since the latter decades of the twentieth century, the body of literature concerned with women and mental health has grown significantly and within which the diverse needs of different groups of women within society have received both increased attention and recognition (Perry 1993, Brockington 1998, Doyal 1998, Ashurst 1999, Smith and Cox 1999, Kohen 2000, Barnes, Davis et al. 2002, Gido and Dalley 2008). In contrast, any specific focus or discussion within the literature concerning the mental health needs or requirements of disabled women who experience mental distress remains small with only a small number of women having published in this area (Begum 1990, 1995, Morris 1991, Keith 1994, Marris 1996, Thomas 1999). In a study which examined the experiences of using mental health services for a group of people with physical impairments living across the UK, (two thirds of whom were women) Morris (2004) drew attention to how needs relating to physical impairment had commonly being unrecognised within mental health services, with some services structurally inaccessible to people with significant mobility impairments due to a failure to comply with the Disability Discrimination Act by making reasonable adjustments. Additionally, poor experiences both of gaining access to, and using community mental health services were reported by individuals with privately funded counselling the sole provision that had been viewed positively (Lonsdale 1990, Morris 2004).

Where the topic area of physical impairment and mental health has, until recent decades, been examined within mental health and psychology literature, the predominant perception of disabled people was for their situation to be characterised by a medically informed personal tragedy perspective (Thomas 1999). Likewise, it was routinely asserted that an individual's disability had likely arisen through his or her circumstances, shortcomings and/or medical condition, with the physical condition viewed as 'a problem for the individual' or as a 'tragedy for which a cure was required' (Fillingham 2012). Within the studies, a clear link has been made between physical impairment and mental health and founded on a premise that a level of depression will automatically be experienced by someone living with a permanent physical impairment. Mostly, two assumptions underpin the literature:

i) that a physical impairment per se is a cause of mental or psychological distress;
ii) that the extent and likelihood of distress, and the solutions to it are to be found within the person.

With studies routinely asking questions such as:

i) Is depression associated with this particular impairment?
ii) What are the factors that make depression more likely?
iii) Does the experience of depression influence the way that impairment is experienced?

Furthermore, much of the literature has suggested that individuals (both women and men) living with a physical impairment will need to make psychological adjustments at a number of stages if they are to fully come to terms with their impairment and to live as a 'psychologically whole being'. A discussion of stage theories and the associated concept of loss will be discussed in more depth within Chapter 3.

Studies which sought to examine a link between living with a physical impairment and experiencing mental distress overwhelmingly assumed the causal link to be found in the experience of impairment per se and the consequential functional limitations, additionally looking at the potential for specific conditions, for example Multiple Sclerosis or Spinal Cord Injury, to impact on mental health and well-being and focusing predominantly on depression as opposed to any other mental health condition (Craig et al. 1997, Kennedy 1999). In a study which examined the incidence of depression among a group of people diagnosed with Multiple Sclerosis (two thirds of whom were women), almost half had experienced a major episode of clinical depression (Sadovnik 1996) whilst Stenager's study (1992) of 50 people living with Multiple Sclerosis discovered high rates of suicide attempts or suicidal ideations when experiencing episodes of decline in functional abilities. Other studies (for example Zarb and Oliver 1987, Craig and Hancock 1997) which identified relatively high rates of depression among physically disabled people, likewise assumed a causal link between an individual's experience of physical impairment and coping with functional limitations but with all having attracted criticism at a number of levels.

Foremost, studies undertaken were criticised for their failure to consider a range of social and economic factors which may accompany, or be associated with physical impairment, such as added financial pressures, potential relationship difficulties and/or the likelihood of temporary or permanent loss of employment for those of a working age. Any potential relevance of factors such as ethnicity, gender or economic and social roles critics claimed to have been considered within only a small number of studies and further drew attention to the lack of consideration given to the disabled person's experience from their personal perspective, which was a fundamental element of my work. An assumption that people living with a physical impairment would experience depression as a response to, or as part of an adjustment to living with their impairment, whilst other forms of mental distress or mental health conditions were seldom considered was further criticised, in addition to the lack of differentiation made when assuming a causal link between individuals born with their impairments, and those who acquired their impairment at some stage during their lives.

The assumption of a causal link has persisted in spite of conflicting evidence both about the co-existence of physical impairment and depression and that existence and degree of depression do not appear to be linked directly to the extent of physical impairment (Morris 2002), and where called into question by the research evidence, some researchers have looked to disabled people's attitudes towards their impairment for an explanation. In an examination of the attitudes of a group of disabled people (women and men) towards their impairments, Leger (2002) concluded that the psychological differences which individuals experienced were neither correlated with degree of impairment nor with whether the impairment was acquired or present from birth, whilst a lower level of acceptance of disability was seen to be significantly associated with more anxious and depressive symptoms. This view was supported by Pilgrim (2005) who claimed that people will differ in their psychological adaptation to losing, or losing the use of limbs, and that whilst some people will develop a prolonged grief reaction to their loss or their individual personality is affected, others will not react in the same way.

Research which has found little correlation between the extent of physical impairment and the level of depression experienced has additionally emphasised the social context of the experience of impairment. For example, Fuhrer's study (1993) which examined incidences of depression among a group of people living with varying levels of functional abilities having acquired spinal cord injuries found there to be no relationship between the two and instead concluding that experiences of depression were associated more with restrictions in social role performance that stemmed from the interactive influences of the environment. Furthermore, in a study which examined the impact on daily life for a group of people living with acquired spinal cord injuries, emphasis was placed on how, in addition to individuals need to maintain their physical health and avoid secondary infections, adjustments often had to be made to family and interpersonal roles. In addition, added financial pressures and a likelihood of temporary or permanent job loss are considered to each have potential to take an emotional toll exceeding that resulting from the sheer magnitude of physical impairment itself (Krause 1997).

In responding to the criticisms levelled at studies undertaken from a medical model perspective, recent decades have witnessed the emergence of studies which in considering the mental health experiences of disabled people (women and men) have adopted a greater social perspective. Such studies, in contrast, began to draw attention to the diversity of factors which disabled people themselves identified as having impacted on (or as having long-term potential to) impact on mental well-being, for example, how the attitudes of able-bodied people towards those who are not can affect self-worth, and how efforts to adopt a positive self-image can be impeded by the devalued status that has historically been ascribed to disabled people. In contrast to the medical model of disability, the literature adopting a social model approach shifts the focus from *impairment* onto *disability*, using the term to refer to disabling social, environmental and attitudinal barriers rather than a lack of physical ability. Similarly, emerging literature began to challenge a prevalent assumption throughout much of the twentieth century that living with a permanent physical disability equated to a life of both poor quality and worth and highlighting its potential to impact on the mental well-being of disabled people (Morris 1991, Vasey 1992). Whilst such experiences have been shown to invoke feelings of anger and rejection amongst disabled people (Campling 1981, Greeley 1996), the psychological consequences of such experiences have yet to be noticeably documented within the literature with the exception of the work of a small minority (for example Thomas 1999, 2004, Reeve 2003, 2004, 2008, 2012) who have called for an extension of the social model of disability which recognises not solely the effect of structural barriers on what disabled people can *do*, but also recognises psycho-emotional disablism and the ways in which this can impact on who disabled people can 'be'. Calls for a renewed social model of disability have also been made over the past two decades by those who consider the original model to be outdated (for example Finkelstein 2001, Shakespeare and Watson 2001) or who wish for a model which includes the personal experience of impairment (Crow 1996) and the arguments for and against which have been, and continue to be, widely debated within disability studies circles and literature. Therefore, whilst my research (Smith 2010) highlighted as one of its key findings the need for teaching around the social model of disability to be widely included within the curriculums of mental health professionals training courses (to be discussed within Chapter 5), in wishing to give a voice to disabled women who have experienced mental distress, the proposed benefits or otherwise of a renewed social model of disability will not be considered within this text.

Living with a Physical Impairment: An Inevitability of Mental Distress?

In seeking to undertake a study which provided a platform for a group of disabled women to share their personal experiences, data evidence demonstrated a range of views expressed in relation to an assumed causal link between living with a physical impairment and experiencing mental distress; whilst six women considered that their impairment or the functional limitations arising from it had been a contributory factor to their experiences of mental distress, six were in disagreement with an assumed causal link. Across the group women recalled experiences of working with mental health professionals within a range of organisations who, relatively early in the working relationship had explained their mental distress as a natural, or to be expected response to living with a physical impairment. In addition, women recalled professionals who considered their impairment to be 'a tragedy' and likewise was viewed as a negative attribute of their persona irrespective of the nature and circumstances surrounding their impairment. However, group-wide none of the women believed their impairment had been either the sole or primary cause of their mental distress, with data evidence consistently reinforcing the perceived vital need for mental health and allied health and social care professionals to recognise the potential of factors other than physical difference and/or functional limitations to impact on mental well-being. Experiences of prolonged hospital stays following the onset of, or linked to a woman's impairment, difficult to control pain, extreme fatigue and reduced energy levels were among a matrix of factors highlighted as having the long-term potential to affect mental well-being with three women having commented on how the combined effects of extreme fatigue and low energy levels could on occasions prove more difficult to cope with than their impairment.

Whether or not some form of mental distress was experienced when living with an impairment (and the acuteness of that distress), was also considered by the majority of women to likely depend on factors such as whether the impairment had been present from birth or had been acquired, and where acquired, whether the onset had been sudden, for example, resulting from a stroke or trauma and/or whether the impairment was of a progressive or unpredictable nature. The likelihood of experiencing a single or repeated episode of mental distress was also considered to be higher amongst women whose physical mobility and/or functional limitations were significantly affected by their impairment and/or where it impacted substantially on daily life and/or physical health.

Where depression or another mental health condition was experienced, there existed a group-wide consensus that, whilst there may be similarities across individuals' experiences of mental distress, ultimately, any experiences will be highly personal to that individual with no uniformed course of treatment or recovery process. Further, women agreed that an individual's reactions to the realisation of a physical impairment being a permanent fixture in their life or responses to the onset of an acquired impairment, may to some degree be determined by an individual's character and personality with any experiences of mental distress possibly linked to what a woman did prior to the onset of impairment for example, their chosen career path, type of employment and/or previous lifestyle.

Two women living with acquired impairments considered the onset of their mental distress had occurred shortly after receiving diagnosis of their medical condition and when confronted with potentially significant life changes. However, their experiences were seen to differ from those of other women with acquired impairments who did not considered themselves to have experienced mental distress until several years after acquiring their impairment. Aged 13 when she acquired a spinal cord injury, Jackie had not felt a need for mental health support until two decades later when she was faced with having to finish work and acknowledged what paid work represented within her daily life:

> When my injury first happened for months after I was upset and a bit down at times but I wouldn't really say depressed and fellow patients on the spinal ward well we all helped each other through the good and not so good days. It wasn't until many years later that I felt mentally I was struggling to cope and needed professional help … but it wasn't about my impairment directly it was more about coming to terms with finishing full time work because of secondary problems linked to my injury which until then I'd managed ok. Going to work five days a week had given a structure to my life and made me feel like a normal person whatever that is … I come from a family who've always worked and after my injury I hadn't wanted to go down the day centre route … I knew my brain needed more than that so I got the best education I could and when faced with finishing work and the stimulation and social contact that came with it I found it tough.
>
> Jackie (age 45, acquired spinal injury)

Amongst the six women living with acquired and/or progressive impairments, four spoke of experiencing episodes of 'if only' days and describing in similar terms living with the constant knowledge that their physical abilities would diminish but with the uncertainty of not knowing when, or at what rate of decline. Women within this group who had experienced repeated episodes of mental distress spoke of subsequent episodes being overall less severe than the preceding one and mostly of a shorter duration, having adjusted to varying extents to their altered life circumstances. During such episodes women similarly recalled periodic yearnings to once again be able to perform independently everyday tasks which previously had been taken for granted, and typically illustrated by Judith who recalled her episodic frustration when unable to perform simple tasks:

> When I came home after my stroke and was adjusting to my changed physical abilities it was the stupid little things like opening a milk carton or picking something up I'd dropped that really got to me ... things that before I wouldn't stop to think about yet now they seemed like big obstacles ... it was the constant having to ask others for help that got me down. Nowadays I've learned all sorts of ways to do things which may not be conventional but work for me ... there's still days when I come up against things at home I can't do but you learn to live with it and just manage the best you can.
>
> Judith (age 61, acquired paralysis following stroke)

A lack of available support and information from health and social care professionals about an individual's specific condition was also highlighted, in particular by women with acquired or progressive impairments and which had led to feelings of isolation. Diagnosed with Multiple Sclerosis in her early thirties, Maria described her feelings of vulnerability in the months post-diagnosis:

> In the months after I was diagnosed all the health people were kind and offered endless cups of tea but what I really needed was facts about the condition and what I should expect to happen or look out for as I knew pretty much nothing. I knew I would probably have to give up full-time work so I needed to know if there were any disability allowances I would be eligible for ... I had three children to feed and clothe but I just recall that with the exception of a few leaflets you were mainly left to your own devices ... Nowadays of course there is the internet where there is a lot of information and advice which wasn't there when I was diagnosed and I felt quite lonely and unsupported at times.
>
> Maria (age 51, acquired neurological impairment)

In a study which examined the daily life experiences of a group of women living with a spinal cord injury (Morris 1989), the lack of concern shown by health and welfare professionals for psychological and emotional needs was highlighted repeatedly by women who were given little space to express their grief during the post injury months. Similarly, women reported receiving little or no help in coming to terms with sudden onset paralysis alongside an expectation to always be smiling and to present as happy and coping. Whilst several women had expressed a wish for counselling, for many it had been the mutually supportive relationships with fellow patients that had made their hospital stays bearable, with criticism levelled at rehabilitation that was perceived to have been too male and sport orientated and which had paid little attention to their specific needs as women. Furthermore, women considered undue emphasis had been placed on regaining the ability to walk whilst conversely little consideration was given to the pain, discomfort and/or fatigue that many women endured post injury and in addition that little assistance with planning for the future had been offered.

The experiences of women with acquired impairments were however shown within my study (Smith 2010) to have differed from those of the women born with their impairments (and which were generally classed as non-progressive such as spina bifida or cerebral palsy) who spoke broadly of having only ever known one level of physical ability. However, this group of women did not wholly consider themselves to be exempt from experiencing mental distress. Whilst they had not had to make adjustments in the way that women with acquired impairments had been required to do (with the exception of physical changes in mobility that were considered to be a natural part of the natural ageing process), each had experienced mental distress and, like the women with acquired impairments had experienced 'if only' days.

Katy, born with brittle bones described a typical 'if only' day:

> I was born with brittle bones and have always used a wheelchair. Growing up I've been through lots of what I call my 'if only' episodes when I've found myself wishing that I could do A, B or C ... They may only be the smallest things or things I've dreamt about or seen people do on the telly ... things I've never experienced and will never get the chance to and it does sadden me but it's the life I have and you do the best you can ... at least my brain is functioning and keeping myself stimulated helps me mentally.
>
> Katy (age 43, congenital impairment)

During these episodes Katy explained how she did not consider herself to be mentally distressed or in need of mental health support but that she experienced a sense of general sadness and group-wide the importance of being able to differentiate between 'feeling a bit down' and suffering from 'real mental distress' which was likely to require professional help was emphasised. Recalling her experience, Frankie highlighted:

> It can be a fine line between what is real depression and what is more a general feeling of being a bit down or low ... but you have to separate the two and be able to recognise true mental distress for the severe illness it can potentially become ... clinical depression left untreated can lead to you becoming mentally quite unwell as I know from experience and I should have sought mental health support much earlier than I did.
>
> Frankie (age 27, congenital impairment)

Attitudes towards Physical Impairment

Evident from women's accounts of their experiences of mental distress, was that to varying degrees the attitudes of other people towards them and/or their impairment had been a factor. In recent decades disabled people have begun to write about difficulties which they have encountered in their everyday contacts with able-bodied people and it has been suggested that interactions between disabled people and able-bodied people often occur in situations in which the former are seen as dependent and negatively different (Robinson, Martin et al. 2007, Crisp 2000).

Further, it has been claimed that the attitudes of able-bodied people towards those who are not can impact on self-image and self-worth (Lonsdale 1990, Lenney and Sercombe 1992, Keith 1996, Collier 1999, Smith 2003). In Morris's (1991) study of the daily life experiences of a group of women living with a spinal cord injury, she argued that it was the attitudes and comments of able-bodied people towards disabled people that made women feel disabled in a way that their impairment did not. One decade later, within a study which examined the meaning of health and disability for a small group of disabled women, Tighe (2010) concluded that the most compelling feature of their narratives had been the pressure to define their health by able-bodied people's standards. Similarly, the women's accounts of their lives, and how they made sense of them, were dominated by a need to struggle against stereotypical social perceptions of disabled people as abnormal, sick and worthy of pity (Tighe 2001).

Writing of her personal experiences of living with an acquired spinal cord injury, Morris (1991) claimed that the attitudes and prejudices of non-disabled people can impact on the lives of disabled people, believing that disabled people have to establish their own values about their lives and insist that non-disabled people recognise these. Furthermore, Morris called for disabled people to be courageous in acknowledging that there are negative things about being disabled as well as the positive things in which disabled people take pride, but that disabled women (and men) must have the ability to define the negative aspects of the experience of disability and *not* the various professionals with whom they may come into contact with. In addition to disabled people often having to deal with the reactions of able-bodied people towards them, Reeve believes that people with visible impairments often have to deal with the curiosity and/or stares of those who may have expectations of how disabled people should 'look' for example, a person of older years sitting in a wheelchair, and which can then cause difficulty for those not fitting the perceived stereotypical image. The experience of being stared at by individuals who may not consider the person to be 'properly disabled', for example, when using a disabled parking space or toilet facilities, Reeve considers to be a potential source of psycho-emotional disablism which can leave disabled people feeling both vulnerable and invalidated (Reeve 2008). Individuals living with less or non-visible impairments may also according to Drewitt (1990) face a battle to be believed and at times find themselves forced to justify a definition of 'disabled' whilst people living with medically unrecognised impairments or conditions are likely to face further challenges;

> Denial of their experience is a major source of loneliness, alienation and despair in people with unrecognised disabilities.
>
> Drewitt 1990: 25

Feelings of vulnerability and invalidation, in particular during 'better days' when her fluctuating impairment was not visibly apparent were talked about by Frankie;

> On what may be a better day, approaching a disabled parking bay at university or the supermarket I find that I'm asking myself should I use the space or not as I know people will look at you and think, there's nothing wrong with her she's walking OK and they'll have a good stare or whisper something under their breath yet I know by parking further away the muscle pain that then may cause and soon a better day becomes anything but … it can leave you feeling very exposed and even self-questioning your impairment which sounds crazy but the way people look at you sometimes it can make you feel like that and I think my young age adds to people's sense of doubting your impairment's validity … that said I think we are making slow progress but there is still some way to go.
>
> Frankie (age 27, congenital impairment)

Born with her hereditary impairment, Lisa also believed that the attitudes of able-bodied people towards her and/or her impairment, in particular during late adolescence had contributed to her mental distress:

> For me the depression seemed to come about in part from the realisation that as I entered into adulthood and became a disabled woman that the world seemed to view me differently than it did able-bodied women. It was as if I wasn't part of normal society and I wasn't sure where I was meant to fit or belong.
>
> Lisa (age 45, congenital impairment)

with similar views expressed by Philippa:

> The depression I've suffered from time to time since my mid-teens has certainly partly been to do with me being disabled but I wouldn't say it's been the primary cause … it's also definitely been about how able-bodied people perceive me as a young disabled woman … maybe not so much now as say 10 or 15 years ago as I have seen changes more recently but I still think that others attitudes towards me as a disabled woman affect me mentally and I have real issues around my self-image.
>
> Philippa (age 36, congenital impairment)

Analysed data further showed a shared belief that historically within society, the existence of both an ignorance of, and a lack of knowledge around physical impairment had resulted from the lack of contact able-bodied people had with people who were not, with societal attitudes towards, and misconceptions held around physical impairment perceived by the majority of women to have been a response to hearsay or what people read about 'disabled people'. Misinformed beliefs such as that disabled people needed to live and/or be cared for within residential institutions, or did not go out to work or live as part of a family unit provoked feelings ranging from irritation to anger with Elisabeth describing the varied emotions she experienced when faced with such assumptions:

> I always remember as a child and in my teens friends of my parents coming to the house for social occasions and their look would always be one of pity and sympathy which hurt me inside … sitting on the stairs when I was meant to be in bed I would hear people asking mum and dad why they didn't look for a home for me so that they didn't have to look after me. I remember dad telling me that soon after I was born the doctor had said the best thing they could do was go home and let the authorities put me in care as they thought it unlikely I would live long and if I did I'd have no quality of life. Well here I am … 62 years of age and going strong so yes that angers me … I just have to convince myself that things are different now or at least I hope so …
>
> Elisabeth (age 62, congenital impairment)

Diagnosed with her impairment during adolescence, Frankie believed the unpredictable nature of her impairment had enabled her to observe any differences in the attitudes of able-bodied people towards her (and her impairment) when not mobilising with a walking aid (and her impairment was not immediately visible) and when mobilising with an aid and her impairment was visibly exposed. Over several years, Frankie recalled her overall experience of people associating a walking aid such as a stick, crutches or frame with a physical impairment and responding accordingly in a sympathetic manner, ever more so if the person was of a young age as opposed to an older person for whom an element of mobility impairment may be anticipated. Whilst group-wide participants had witnessed a positive shift in attitudes towards physical impairment over recent decades, and particularly since entering the new millennium, there remained group-wide a belief in the continuing existence of a credibility gap between *visible* and *non-visible* impairments with a perception that people were overall more 'believing' of the former rather than the latter. Further, women believed there to now exist within society a greater general awareness and understanding of issues around visible physical impairments as opposed to those which are less or not visible, and whilst such greater awareness and understanding was welcomed, there was unanimous agreement of the need to not become complacent and of the scope that remained for ongoing improvement.

As the youngest participant, Carly considered herself fortunate to have been educated during an era when positive shifts in attitudes towards disabled people and disability generally were occurring across society. During her primary education in the early twenty-first century, Carly encountered no problems with attitudes towards her impairment, having often been a source of entertainment among classmates who took turns to push her around the playground in her wheelchair. In contrast, on moving to secondary school Carly had become self-conscious of her impairment;

> When I moved to mainstream secondary my peers were of an age where they were very self-conscious of who they were seen with or made friends with and

> it took a while to make friends which was hard as I hadn't experienced that in primary school from boys or girls ... I think for a lot of people it was about the wheelchair as historically that seems to have symbolised physical disability ... disabled parking spaces ... disabled toilets ... access signs ... they all use wheelchair logos and people associate it with someone who is badly disabled and helpless and they're initially anxious as it's the first thing they see. I think if I'd been on crutches or walking sticks that sense of reluctance to mix with you wouldn't have been so noticeable but it felt like the chair was a large, visible barrier between you and them.
>
> Carly (age 18, congenital impairment)

Carly's experience however, contrasted markedly with that of Jackie who, in the late 1970s acquired a spinal cord injury shortly after starting secondary school. Later resuming her education within a special school environment, Jackie had been pleasantly surprised to find herself still welcomed among her previous circle of able-bodied friends who endeavoured to include her wherever possible within their out of school activities to shopping centres, cinemas etc. despite the structural barriers to access which in the early 1980s were then commonplace. These two contrasting experiences, Jackie attributed to a belief of her impairement having been acquired during an era when adolescents were much less image conscious than those of today's world who are incessantly subjected through diverse media forms to images of so-called perfect-looking body shapes, targeted particularly at adolescents and young women, a theme of which shall be discussed in more depth elsewhere.

For Judith, following a stroke which had resulted in substantially reduced mobility, no significant problems with people's attitudes towards herself or her impairment had been encountered (in contrast to the attitudes of some people previously known to her and to be discussed later in this chapter) which she attributed partly to the relative invisibility of her impairment to others following intensive rehabilitation. However, Jackie believed that her experiences may have been altered if her speech had been affected;

> After my stroke I spent four months on the stroke rehab ward and there were people at different stages in their recovery ... as a group of patients we tried to support each other and other patients relatives would stop by and have a chat. it became almost like a second family ... but it was quite noticeable how people whose speech had been affected tended to be overlooked and almost became isolated which I found sad as that could've been me. I think people were unsure how to speak to someone who was having problems communicating verbally but I just did my best to talk to anyone affected ... the same way as I would to anyone else.
>
> Judith (age 61, acquired paralysis following stroke)

Throughout her stay on a rehabilitation ward with patients who, like herself, had acquired a mobility impairment as a result of stroke or spinal injury, Judith recalled her observations of people initially being unwilling to use a wheelchair for fear of it representing the labelling of themselves as a 'disabled person' and as it having a stigma attached to it but that visitors to the ward would respond with sympathy and kindness to any wheelchair-user patients.

Accessing the Environment

In addition to the diverse ways in which women had experienced the attitudes of others towards them and/or their impairment, a prolonged inability to access public buildings and arenas was also identified as an additional factor which, in the long term, women felt had the potential to affect mental well-being (Barnes 1991). The improvements in structural access which had steadily taken place through the latter decades of the twentieth century, and in particular following implementation of the Disability Discrimination Act (1995), had been welcomed group-wide for removing many of the physical barriers which historically had prevented access to public spaces and buildings for disabled people, in particular those with significant mobility impairments and wheelchair users. The dismantling of barriers and subsequent improved access to the environment was unanimously believed to have positively affected mental well-being through creating a sense of feeling more integrated within a society that was beginning to acknowledge their access requirements as disabled women. In particular, they were welcomed by women who had lived through decades when access and opportunities to interact socially within public social spaces had been severely hampered (Barnes 2011). Furthermore, most women believed that an increased visibility of disabled women (and men) within society had led to able-bodied people having more interaction with disabled people than in previous decades, when significant numbers of the disabled population resided within long-stay hospitals or residential institutions and were rarely seen in public arenas. These women recalled having grown up being excluded from a society which catered only for the needs of a majority able-bodied population and with limited opportunities to access higher education or meaningful employment. Improved structural access had subsequently resulted in openings for disabled people to pursue higher education or employment with opportunities to work alongside able-bodied colleagues as opposed to working within specialised workshops for disabled people where menial work was undertaken in return for a small wage which UK-wide had hitherto been commonplace.

Self-image and Mental Well-being

In addition to examining the impact of societal attitudes towards physical impairment on mental well-being, the study sought women's views with regard to whether attitudes towards impairment were felt to have the potential to affect the self-image of disabled women, and if so, then to what extent. In examining the psycho-emotional impact of living as a disabled person Reeve (2008, 2013) drew attention to the issue of internalised oppression which occurs when a marginalised group in society (disabled people) internalises the prejudices held by the dominant group (able-bodied people). This oppression is described by Morris (1991) as the acceptance and incorporation of 'their values about our lives', with this form of oppression being most effective when acting at the subconscious level and affecting the self-esteem of the individual in addition to shaping their thoughts and actions (Marks 1999). Whilst over recent decades increasing numbers of disabled people have spoken about the disabling attitudes they experience in their daily lives, Marks (1999) claimed there had been scant recognition within the mental health or disability studies literature of either the feelings of anger or distress potentially evoked by such attitudes, or of the short- or long-term psychological consequences of such experiences, but each being topic areas that my research was keen to explore.

Group-wide, analysed data demonstrated a firm belief that the attitudes of able-bodied people towards impairment, combined with the devalued status commonly ascribed within society to disabled people, and which to some degree was felt to still exist, could impede on women's efforts to adopt a positive self-image. Likewise, historical assumptions both within society and amongst medical professionals that living a life with a physical impairment equated to a life lacking worth or quality many women felt had the long-term potential to affect mental well-being (Basnett 1992, Shakespeare 1994). Evidenced by the data and of noteworthy interest was the prevalence of poor self-image amongst women in the upper age ranges, and in particular amongst women born with their impairments with Elisabeth one of four women who, whilst growing up had considered themselves inferior to able-bodied people;

> Well, growing up you didn't see people like me out in public places … so it felt that to be like me must be a negative thing and that I wasn't the sort of person people would really want to get to know or to come into contact with in the outside world.
>
> Elisabeth (age 62, congenital impairment)

Further evidenced by the data was the importance that women attached to having a positive self-image, with several describing their efforts to 'look smart' or 'dress nicely' as attempts to 'feel like other women' whilst simultaneously providing a confidence boost when in public arenas and situations where able-bodied, 'normal' women were present. For two women, their poor self-image had been compounded by their communication difficulties, with Helen additionally perceiving herself to have been a burden on her family throughout her pre-adult years:

> We were quite a large family and maybe a few times a year on special occasions we would go out together for something to eat … 30 years ago finding a family restaurant that had wheelchair access wasn't easy so I always felt like an obstacle being hauled up steps and attracting people's attention as they moved chairs to make way for you and gave pitiful glances … often I felt in the way and that I'd

> only been brought along as I couldn't be left at home ... I would go to speak and mum would look at me as if to say please don't Helen so as not to bring attention to me ... that's really stuck with me and a general sense of feeling unloved which has affected my self-image and self-worth ... even now in my forties.
>
> Helen (age 41, congenital impairment)

Helen's experience contrasted with those of other women for whom both maintaining a positive self-image whilst resisting pressure to conform to 'normality' was considered important, with Elisabeth recalling the changes she had observed over recent decades in relation to expectations of conformity and social norms:

> When I lived at home until I was about 30 we always did our annual family holiday to the seaside which brought its challenges given the lack of access that existed then generally but as a treat we would eat out in cafes a couple of times ... my misplaced joints meant holding a knife and fork was really hard and I had my own way of holding them differently which mum accepted at home but in public she insisted I behaved 'normally' despite it being painful. Over time I got weary of being expected to conform to able-bodied norms and decided I wasn't doing it any more. Three decades on and it's a relief that there's greater awareness and now I do things in a way that works for me and if anyone has a problem with it well too bad. I think in that respect events such as the Paralympics has shown that people can do things whether it be sports or other stuff just as well as able-bodied people, it's just that they achieve things in a different way.
>
> Elisabeth (age 62, congenital impairment)

Highlighted within the women's accounts was the significant role felt to have been played by the media in affecting self-image. Clearly evidenced by the study data were the widely expressed feelings of dissatisfaction and frustration concerning the historical portrayal within the media of disabled people as either heroes, of having achieved some amazing feat or as charitable cases or victims worthy of pity and sympathy, thus presenting both inaccurate and unrealistic accounts of how the majority of disabled women (and men) live their daily lives (Sancho 2003). Through presenting the lived experiences of disabled people in such a negative way, attention was similarly drawn by Barnes (1991) to the ways in which the media had for too long done too little in assisting to improve attitudes towards, or increasing awareness of physical impairment and disability within society.

However, apparent from both the analysed data and the literature that was beginning to examine whether or not the introduction of anti-discrimination legislation had affected the lives of disabled people and if so, then in what ways, was a recognition that the latter years of the twentieth- and the start of the twenty-first century had seen gradual changes taking place in relation to the improved portrayal of disability and impairment within diverse media realms.

There had also been an observable increase in the presence of disabled people and characters on television, in film, the arts and in the press, with the television coverage of the 2012 Paralympics felt to have been particularly influential (Imrie 2004, Day 2005, Hurstfield and Meager 2006). This topic will be examined further in a later chapter. Whilst such changes had been broadly welcomed, some forms of the media were still considered to be doing little to promote positive disability awareness. In particular, the content of women's fashion and beauty magazines were continuing to affect women's self-worth and image through repeated use of supposedly perfect-looking, able-bodied women which, combined with a virtual or total absence of disabled women reinforced their sense of not being 'normal'. However, group-wide there was recognition that the use of supposed perfect-looking models (which are now commonly digitally enhanced using airbrushed techniques) in publications aimed at a young female audience have over recent years attracted wide criticism from a number of concerned organisations for the role they are perceived to play in impacting on the self-image of able-bodied teenage girls and young women and that it was not an issue of concern solely for disabled women.

Physical Impairment and Relationships

In addition to attracting criticism for their lack of attention paid to social factors which critics believed had the potential to affect mental well-being and which have been examined above, studies which suggested a causal link between living with a physical impairment and experiencing mental distress were further criticised for the lack of consideration paid to the impact of a person's physical impairment upon their relationships with spouses, partners, family, friends or significant persons within their life. Likewise, the topic of disabled people and their relationships with family, friends or significant persons in their lives has not been widely discussed. Based upon the research evidence, the final part of this chapter will therefore consider the impact of living with a physical impairment upon women's relationships with significant others in their life and within the context of their experiences of mental distress.

Family Relationships

Whilst family may be a source of support to some individuals adjusting and/or adapting to changed circumstances, with their impairment becoming an integral part of family life (in instances where an impairment is acquired), for others the reaction of family members to physical impairment may cause distress and/or upset if their impairment is perceived to be something that has caused disruption to family life (Morris 1991, Thomas 1998, Smith 2003). Whilst some women believed their impairment had contributed to their experience of mental distress, unanimously the women believed that any likelihood of experiencing mental distress may, to some degree be determined by the relationships individuals had with significant people within their lives. The importance of having ready access to support networks which provided both practical and emotional support at times of need were considered to be crucial to the process of adjustment to impairment, in particular where an impairment had been acquired through illness or sudden onset trauma, and following which individuals may be faced with major changes and significant upheaval within their lives.

The relationships which women had with family members were shown by the research evidence to have varied widely: whilst some women with acquired impairments recalled immediate family members struggling to come to terms with the person's diagnosis, others spoke of family members who, from the time of diagnosis or when their impairment was acquired, had provided support and encouragement in helping them to adjust both to their changed physical abilities and life circumstances. The dynamics of family relationships for women with acquired impairments (in particular two women with impairments acquired as adolescents) were also shown to have differed in a number of ways from those of women with congenital impairments. After sustaining a spinal cord injury when aged 13, the support and encouragement provided by Jackie's parents enabled her to rebuild her life, with her altered physical abilities being integrated into the family's daily life. Conversely, Jackie's spinal injury had been viewed by her grandparents as 'a tragedy' which, Jackie perceived to be a reflection of the era in which they had grown up and when large numbers of disabled people lived within residential institutions and attracted pity from the able-bodied outside world. Having also acquired a spinal illness in her teens, Claire recalled the overwhelming support of some family members who had rallied around whilst others had struggled to cope with her changed circumstances and reacted by avoiding face-to-face contact:

> The first few months I was unwell the family all rallied around but as time went on and it was clear my paralysis was going to be permanent there were family [members] who were more accepting and others who couldn't really cope and dealt with it by staying away and not really having contact. It was just their way of dealing with it but even today there are family who are more comfortable with you than others … they'll talk to you on the phone as that way they don't actually have to see you in a wheelchair in person or have to do anything to help physically …
>
> Claire (aged 39, acquired spinal illness)

Diagnosed with Multiple Sclerosis in her early thirties, at that time a mother to three young children, Maria recalled her husband's difficulty in coming to terms with her diagnosis. In endeavouring to maintain a positive and strong approach for her family, Maria found herself left with little opportunity to express her own feelings about her changed life circumstances:

> When I'd been for a few tests throughout I'd convinced myself it was something trivial so the diagnosis of MS came as a huge shock … I didn't know much about it but knew it wasn't a nice illness. I struggled to come to terms with it and my husband took it really badly and the kids had to be told something though they were too young to fully understand … Seeing my husband so sad was tough … he just felt helpless and I had to be the strong one who kept things together which left little time for my own thoughts and over time things built up and it did affect me mentally and affected us as a family in different ways.
>
> Maria (age 51, acquired neurological impairment)

Women with congenital impairments who were also the eldest, or one of the elder family siblings were seen to have experienced relatively few problems with family relationships during their childhood years. With recollections similar to those of two fellow participants, Katy described how siblings questioning about her 'physical difference' had been honestly answered by her parents using age-appropriate language, which had resulted in her differences being readily accepted and integrated within the family unit. Other women born with their impairments described relationship difficulties with their parents at different stages of their growing up; whilst some women considered their parents to have been over-protective and had neither involved nor enabled the woman to take responsibility about decisions in her pre-adult life, others recalled having been treated differently and shown less love than their siblings which had contributed to periodic episodes of emotional distress. As the first-born to a farming family, Alison believed the fact she was a girl, *and* born with spina bifida had been a double disappointment to her father, and upon learning during early adolescence that her father had wanted as his first-born a son who could continue to work the farm in the years ahead, had permanently affected her daughter/father relationship. Furthermore, Alison recalled how the lack of love shown by her father when growing up had led her to marry at the early age of 19, but that the tensions created by relatives had led to her marriage break-up after just four years:

> I always felt my in-laws considered me second best … Rick had mobility problems but didn't use a wheelchair like me … we'd been at school together for many years and I thought it was true love even though I was still young … I think the in-laws felt their son could have done better by marrying an able-bodied woman and all I ever heard from them was negativity and how life would become more difficult as I got older because I was in a wheelchair … it really ground me down and did nothing for my self-image which hit rock bottom and it soon became clear our marriage had little chance of surviving … it was very sad.
>
> Alison (age 38, congenital impairment)

As one of six siblings, Helen had for many years considered herself a burden to her family and, despite a close bond with an elder sibling, believed it to have been her sense of growing up feeling unloved which had led to the onset of psychological difficulties during her teens which had continued into adulthood and beyond. Despite negative perceptions of her childhood and young adult life, Helen spoke of feeling no resentment towards her parents and was one of three women who, on becoming adults, became acutely aware of the lack of practical support and information that had been available to parents of a disabled child during the mid-twentieth century, and of the likely strain this would have placed on parents, especially when there were siblings to care for.

Whilst the women had been greatly appreciative of parents and other family members who, for some women, had provided the practical care and support they required over several decades (and continued to do so), a minority of women recalled occasions when the emotional support they were needing or seeking had been lacking. Elisabeth described her experience:

> When I went through investigations for breast cancer a few years ago I was really anxious as I'd had treatment some years earlier and was worried sick it had returned and felt I needed some emotional support from family … someone just to hold my hand but it just wasn't there … I felt I'd always been there for family at any time of crisis or when any help was needed and it did affect my relationship with them for quite a while though I don't recall us sitting down and resolving things.
>
> Elisabeth (age 62, congenital impairment)

Similarly, Carly recalled her parents struggle to understand her emotional distress following complex surgery linked to her impairment:

> After my surgery I was very low for quite a while and would get very tearful as I felt so helpless and vulnerable but Mum and Dad didn't seem to know what to do for the best and I got frustrated as to be honest neither did I.
>
> Carly (age 18, congenital impairment)

However, among the group there was agreement that, whereas practical support was more tangible and easier to define – for example someone's physical care needs – emotional and psychological needs were harder to define and that, to an extent, all parties had been unsure of how to deal with the situation and circumstances with which they were faced.

Physical Impairment and Friendships

Within the context of their experiences of living as disabled women, the importance and value of friendships have been documented within the literature, and analysed data demonstrated diverse experiences of friendships for both women with congenital impairments and those with acquired impairments and with differences also evident across age spectrums. Within a text of narratives of the daily lives of a group of disabled women, Keith (1994) evidenced how the reactions of friends to physical impairment could vary widely, in particular in situations where impairments had been acquired, and more so when acquired during adolescence or as a younger adult. Whilst for a minority of women relationships with friends had been strengthened after acquiring their impairment, many had witnessed friends distancing themselves which commonly was attributed to friends being unsure of how to react to a friend's changed physical appearance and/or functional abilities with such experiences routinely described as being emotionally hurtful and as having impacted negatively on self-image. The findings from Keith's (1994) study were disappointingly mirrored within a small study one decade later (Smith 2003) in which, amongst other topics, eight disabled women described the impact of living with a physical impairment upon their friendships, with seven having recalled changed friendship dynamics either after acquiring their impairment or following a decline in their physical condition.

Recent study data further evidenced how both age, and the era during which women grew up, had been significant factors within women's overall experiences of friendships. Women who had grown up during the mid-twentieth century when the environment was mostly inaccessible to individuals with mobility impairments recalled difficulties in making friendships throughout their childhood and entering into adulthood, contrasting with the experiences of younger women who entered adulthood at a time when structural barriers were slowly being eroded and the environment was steadily becoming more accessible to disabled people, thereby providing increased opportunities to socialise in public arenas and subsequently enabling greater possibilities of forming friendships. For women in the higher age ranges, efforts to build lasting friendships were consistently considered to have been affected by the historical negative attitudes towards physical impairment which had been prevalent within society throughout their childhood and younger adulthood, changes in which had slowly become evident over recent years and which for younger women especially were considered to now increasingly be enabling disabled women (and men) more opportunities to forge friendships with disabled and non-disabled people alike.

Two women acquired their impairments as young adolescents during the same year (1979), yet their experiences of the reactions of their respective friends to the onset of impairment had contrasted widely and with different explanations offered for its occurrence by each of the women. For Jackie, sustaining friendships after acquiring her spinal cord injury, which occurred during an era when disabled people were seldom seen in public places, had not been experienced as problematic, with friends known to her prior to her injury showing neither discomfort or embarrassment when spending time with a young severely-disabled person in a wheelchair. Additionally, Jackie recalled her parents' role in ensuring that her pre-injury friendships were maintained by amongst other things encouraging friends to share any concerns or ask any questions about Jackie's injury, all of which were answered honestly and in so doing allayed any possible fears or anxieties.

In contrast, following her spinal illness diagnosis Claire had endured a prolonged hospital admission which, friends had associated with recovery and had therefore possibly being confused by Claire's lack of physical progress. Additionally, Claire believed the sudden onset of her paralysis may have created anxieties for her friends about their own vulnerability and they had been wary of asking questions, thus distancing themselves had possibly been considered the easiest option:

> When I was first in hospital friends visited all the time but soon it became clear that I wasn't going to recover and go back to school, to my friends and how things were before ... they didn't quite know what to say or how to react and gradually over time with the exception of one or two friends they stopped coming. I remember being really upset but over time I came to realise that they were just young girls like me and they couldn't understand what was happening any more than I could.
>
> Claire (age 39, acquired spinal illness)

Within the context of her experiences of friendships, Jackie considered the age at which she acquired her impairment to have been a factor, believing that if her injury had occurred 10 years later then both the experiences of those friendships and their dynamics may have been altered. Jackie considered that people in their early twenties would likely have matured into young adults and would have felt less comfortable lifting her from a wheelchair to carry her upstairs, or sit alongside them on grass in the way that both she and her young teenage friends had then felt at ease with.

Women with acquired and/or progressive impairments recollected friends who had drifted away either in the months following the onset of impairment or, during or after a decline in their physical abilities, whilst some women had lost friendships when the commonality upon which they had been founded was lost, for example, friendships made within the workplace. In instances where friends had stayed loyal, women emphasised the positive effect on their mental well-being through the feeling it created of 'belonging' within a circle of friends, and of feeling the same person they had been prior to the onset of impairment but with altered physical abilities.

Maria described her upset when witnessing long-standing friends having decreasing contact as her physical abilities lessened and her speech became affected. Additionally, her upset had been further compounded by a sense of increased isolation resulting from having to leave a job in which for two decades she had been happy and fulfilled and which had enabled social contact with colleagues and the general public alike. However, Maria remained greatly appreciative of a small number of friends who, throughout the highs and lows of her condition had consistently provided support on a number of levels, a sentiment that was mirrored by other women who likewise appreciated 'true friends' who saw them foremost as a person and not as someone defined primarily by their physical impairment.

Further evidenced by the study were the particular difficulties experienced in forming friendships for women who attended special schools and had seldom been provided with opportunities to socialise outside of school, due in part to the large geographical areas from which they drew and to a lack of accessible public transport through many decades of the twentieth century. Educated for 11 years within special schools, Katy described the barriers she encountered in making friends throughout this time:

> This big bus would pull up outside my house emblazoned with [the] 'school for the handicapped' logo in huge letters, you would pick up fellow pupils but you couldn't really talk to people as you'd be locked down in your chair and your so-called friend would be three rows behind you … the same thing every afternoon and so on … pupils came from miles around so you rarely saw people outside of school and even if you'd wanted to public transport wasn't accessible then … neither were there the wheelchair accessible vehicles that are available today … Plus, there was no mobile phones or internet three decades ago, it was a different era … things have changed so much and now in my forties with better access to places and also technology I've more friends than I've ever had.
>
> Katy (age 43, congenital impairment)

Also recalled by a number of women were break times at school having regularly been allocated to physiotherapy or hydrotherapy or personal care needs which consequently allowed little leisure time with fellow pupils. Likewise, for other women, regular hospital admissions for treatment or surgery which were linked to their condition, and were often followed by long periods of recovery at home, had restricted their opportunities to make lasting friendships. Claire recalled long admissions to children's wards where the minority of patients of a similar age had often either been too unwell to form friendships with, or upon discharge home did not maintain contact despite promises to do so. Transferring to a residential home for disabled adults after a long-awaited hospital discharge, Claire encountered few opportunities to form friendships with residents of a similar age due to age differences, and her ability to enter into a relationship with a fellow resident was affected by the lack of privacy afforded to residents:

> There'd been a chap at the special school I had gone to who just happened to live at the residential home and we'd become good friends at school and got to sometimes spend time together during the day at the home but it was really difficult to have any boyfriend–girlfriend relationship as there was so little privacy … because of our care needs you couldn't spend any time together without everyone knowing about it plus it was a home rule that relationships between residents weren't allowed. A few years later he moved out to his own place with care support as he wanted more independence and privacy and really wanted to have a normal relationship … we were together for quite some time and carers gave us privacy realising we were two responsible consenting adults but sadly his health declined and he passed away far too young, I was devastated.
>
> Claire (age 39, acquired spinal illness)

Whilst women educated within special or boarding school environments had experienced barriers to forming friendships, those who attended residential colleges of Further Education for disabled students had encountered fewer difficulties. Lisa described how three years spent within a fully accessible environment had provided numerous opportunities to forge friendships, a view shared by other women who were able to access further or, more latterly, higher education. However, a point stressed by all women was how the common thread of being physically impaired did not constitute making automatic friendships and that they were forged in the same way as able-bodied people formed friendships such as having things in common, similar hobbies or interests, or similar personalities.

Additionally, the diverse forms of technology, communication and social media forums that in the early twenty-first century are now commonplace, and upon which friendships are commonly now made and maintained, had not been available for most of the twentieth century and subsequently restricted the forging of friendships for disabled people. In addition, for three women, difficulties in forming friendships were described as having been compounded by barriers to verbal communication. Whilst the rapid advances in information technology within recent decades were believed to have been instrumental in reducing or eliminating some of the historical barriers to forging and maintaining friendships, such advances were perceived to have been mainly within the home realm for example, through internet forums and social networking sites and were felt not to equate with face to face contact with friends within social settings. Helen's views were echoed by two fellow participants who relied on both verbal and non-verbal means of communication:

> Certainly, advances in technology mean that I can sit in front of my adapted computer and talk to friends online using my keyboard and webcam but it's not the same as meeting up for a coffee or having a bite to eat with a friend in a social place where there's the atmosphere of others around. With the social networks and using the camera once the computer is off that's it you're back to being home on your own and you can still feel isolated. Now places are more accessible I can go out but generally it's with my PAs as I am self-conscious of my speech difficulties and you see the embarrassment on people's faces when they can't understand you so often they stay away rather than trying to understand.
>
> Helen (age 41, congenital impairment)

Physical Impairment and Personal Relationships

Finally, in considering the topic of personal relationships, analysed data likewise highlighted diverse experiences with the difficulties experienced by three women in the late 1980s/early 1990s in seeking heterosexual relationships widely attributed to societal attitudes towards impairment that prevailed throughout much of the twentieth century. Elisabeth's experience mirrored closely that of two other women who during this period approached mainstream dating agencies:

> I made enquiries at a few dating agencies and they took all the basic details but when I mentioned my disability I was met each time with a terrible response … they said they couldn't see how an able-bodied man would want to have a friendship or relationship with a woman who was severely disabled and yet these people hadn't even met me … personality or other attributes didn't seem to matter … They suggested a dating agency for disabled people would be more appropriate which I didn't think even existed then. I'd been married 20 years earlier to a wonderful, able-bodied wonderful man and I recall then people assuming he was my carer … I'd thought things would have moved on then but sadly it seemed not and it really knocked my confidence.
>
> Elisabeth (age 62, congenital impairment)

The responses encountered by each woman had affected both their self-image and overall mental well-being and whilst all had observed notable changes in attitudes towards disability in general since their negative experiences, each had at a later date opted to use dating agencies for disabled people as opposed to mainstream agencies and which for two women had led to successful long-term relationships.

For other women, to varying extents their impairment was considered to have been significant within the context of their relationships with their spouse/partner; whilst six women were not currently in relationships (information which was not requested but offered voluntarily), three stated this to currently be through choice. Judith spoke of being married for 19 years when she suffered her stroke and that her resulting impairment had affected her relationship with her husband:

> After I had my stroke my husband was very supportive and helped me greatly through the initial months but it was further down the line the problems started … niggly things which just then escalated and eventually we separated … looking back now it was all linked to having the stroke and I think if it weren't for that we'd still be together and it is sad as I think it comes back to there being such little support after stroke for the person themselves and those closest to them … I've been on my own now for a while and think I'm better that way … I think it takes a certain type of person to be in a relationship with someone with a physical impairment and I don't want that upset again.
>
> Judith (age 61, acquired paralysis following stroke)

Two women with acquired impairments who were married with children described their acquired impairments as having brought challenges at a number of levels to their relationship, but spoke of the love and support of their spouses having enabled their marriages to remain intact. Of the remaining three women, Frankie was in a long-term relationship with a partner whom she considered to have a good understanding and awareness of her fluctuating condition and that talking through any difficulties she experienced such as physical pain or feeling down was a key element to their strong relationship. Both Lisa and Alison were in long-term relationships with partners who themselves had a physical impairment and their mutual understanding and awareness of each other's circumstances had been vital in sustaining their lasting relationships.

Conclusions

Within this chapter three areas have been considered. Firstly, it has examined the long-held assumed causal link within medical and psychology bodies of literature between living with a physical impairment and experiencing mental distress, and considered its problematic nature through illustrating the diverse factors which within the research were considered to have the potential to impact on the mental well-being of disabled women as opposed to a sole focus on an individual's impairment per se. Issues such as societal attitudes towards impairment, an ability or otherwise to access the outside world and women's self-image were each highlighted as factors of relevance, whilst women's physical impairments per se, whether it had been present from birth or been acquired and the era during which women grew up were shown to be relevant within the context of women's overall life experiences. The chapter has further discussed women's perspectives on whether living with impairment had impacted on their relationships with families, spouses, partners and friends. Both a witnessed shift in areas such as societal attitudes towards physical impairment and disabled people themselves, and an improved awareness and understanding of both disability and impairment were considered to have been relevant within how women experienced their relationships with others.

Having examined women's views relating to an inevitability of mental distress and factors which were felt to have affected their mental well-being, Chapter 2 will now examine women's experiences of gaining access to, and using, mental health service provision.

Chapter 2
Accessing and Using Mental Health Services

Introduction

Within the limited literature which, to date, has examined the topic area of mental health provision for disabled people in the UK who experience mental distress (women and men), it has shown how historically barriers to access have emerged before a counselling relationship could be established due to inaccessible buildings, communication barriers or a lack of information for people from different ethnic backgrounds and cultures (Pelletier 1989, Begum 1999). Likewise, where disabled adults have managed to access services, overwhelmingly the process has been shown to be one fraught with difficulties, with service provision predominantly considered to have been inappropriate for individual's needs (Smith 2003). In a recent study which examined mental health provision within England and Wales for people with physical impairments, the many difficulties which individuals had encountered in locating an accessible therapist or counsellor were highlighted, along with evidence of examples relating to direct service provision where there had been a failure to comply with the Disability Discrimination Act by making reasonable adjustments (Morris 2004). Working with the detailed study findings, this chapter will focus on the findings relating to women's experiences of accessing mental health services across both the statutory and non-statutory sector over a time span of approximately four decades before proceeding to examine women's experiences of using services that were accessed.

Access to Mental Health Services

Within the context of the women's experiences of mental distress, the research study sought to determine whether a shared set of barriers currently existed both in relation to accessing and using mental health services across both the statutory and non-statutory sector. Highlighted clearly within a large majority of the women's accounts were examples of the diverse barriers that had been encountered in endeavouring to access mental health support and/or treatment such as difficulties in accessing relevant information and long waiting times to access services, with differences in experiences also evident amongst women who endeavoured to access provision within the statutory, non-statutory or private sectors. Likewise, analysed data demonstrated differences in experiences between women who sought support during the mid-twentieth century when availability of community-based services were generally limited. In instances where they did exist, locations had overwhelmingly been structurally inaccessible to people with physical impairments whose mobility was significantly affected, whilst those who sought support post-implementation of the Disability Discrimination Act (1995), following which service providers became legally required to provide for the access (and other) requirements of people with physical (and visual and sensory) impairments, reported less barriers to access.

Structural Barriers to Access

Endeavours to access mental health support and/or the treatment that was required, had for several women been hindered at an early stage by physical barriers, for example, steps located at entrances to, or within, buildings where services were located or a lack of accessible transport to reach service locations. In particular, structural barriers had been problematic for older women within the sample group who had sought mental health support prior to the introduction of anti-discrimination legislation when service providers had no legal obligation to meet the access requirements of disabled people. Katy's experience in the early 1980s was echoed by three other women:

> After my dad died I spent time in the residential home as mum couldn't really manage and I was really low ... eventually the doctor at the home said they would arrange some counselling for me. It seemed like I waited ages but then when I went by ambulance it was miles away and based within an old psychiatric hospital and the counsellor worked in an upstairs attic room that was totally inaccessible. They offered to carry me and my electric chair up four flights of stairs but with my brittle bones there was no way I would agree to that. In the end their solution was to see you on one of the ward day rooms but being the place it was mentally unwell patients wandered in and out which was quite scary and there was no privacy. The combination of that and the long journey just added to my depression and in the end I gave up going ... it was doing more harm than good.
>
> Katy (age 43, congenital impairment)

In addition to accessibility issues, Alison's rural home location had meant that travelling times frequently exceeded that allocated to her counselling sessions:

> In the early eighties I had no access to my own transport and public transport wasn't wheelchair accessible so was reliant on NHS transport – of course they don't offer exact times and often by the time you arrived half of your allocated time had gone but the session couldn't be extended as the next person was waiting. You could then wait an hour or so to be taken home and it was just disheartening ... it just felt nothing was being achieved and by the time my sessions ended I didn't feel I was any better mentally than when I started ... it was a real disappointment as I'd set my hopes on it helping.
>
> Alison (age 38, congenital impairment)

Within the sample group, only one woman had received in-patient psychiatric care within five locations across the UK and with access difficulties having been encountered in all but one admission. During Claire's first admission in the late 1980s to a unit within a long-stay Victorian hospital, ward staff had no previous experience of caring for a wheelchair-user patient and adaptations needed to be made before her reluctant admission could take place. Subsequent admissions, all of which occurred after the introduction of the Disability Discrimination Act (DDA 1995) and within newly built constructions, still failed to cater for the physical access needs of individuals with significant mobility impairments, thus reinforcing Claire's increasing concerns over a perceived stark polarisation of services for physically disabled people and those with mental health difficulties.

Such experiences were however seen to contrast with those of other women for whom access issues had not been overly problematic, having sought mental health support post implementation of the Disability Discrimination Act (DDA 1995) and following which service providers were legally obliged to meet the access and other requirements of people with physical (and visual and sensory) impairments. Having accessed counselling in the early twenty-first century, Jackie also considered herself fortunate to have received support at a time when shifts away from hospital-based treatment to community-based services were taking place, whilst her ability to forge a good rapport with the female counsellor with relative ease Jackie believed had contributed to a positive experience of receiving support which had been effective in addressing issues linked to her mental distress:

> When I went to my GP last year I felt really low having had to finish working in a job I enjoyed. We have a good relationship and he knows I only ask for something if I really need it ... he knew I was struggling to cope so said he would arrange some counselling ... I expected to wait ages as I'd heard all sorts of nightmare stories about long waiting times and imagined I'd have to travel the other side of the city ... I was really surprised when someone called within a week of referral and offering an appointment at my local health centre which was nearby and fully wheelchair accessible so that took some of the stresses away.
>
> Jackie (age 45, acquired spinal cord injury)

The ability to access counselling services within locations that catered both for their access and other requirements (reserved disabled parking spaces, accessible toilet facilities and comfortable seating of a manageable height) were also welcomed by two women who accessed counselling support within their respective educational institutions with relative ease. The ability to self-refer to their university support services was considered by both women to have minimised the wait for an initial assessment of their needs which had taken place within two weeks of their respective self-referrals, and in turn was felt to have minimised the risk of their mental distress becoming more acute whilst waiting to have their needs assessed.

Having developed symptoms of anxiety and depression in the months after moving away from home to study, Carly recalled her experience:

> When I first moved away from home to go to college I was excited but nervous as well as it was such a long way and I was only 17 … I hadn't envisaged how homesick I'd be and over the weeks got really anxious and then really down and realised I needed to talk to someone. Fortunately, I'd chosen the college partly because of its good access so knew where counselling support was located was accessible but worried about waiting times so when I found out you could self-refer that was a real help … I think I only waited a couple of weeks to get an appointment which I was so grateful for and with weekly sessions with the counsellor a few months later I was mentally a lot better.
>
> Carly (age 18, congenital impairment)

Access to Information

Research undertaken by the Office of Disability Studies (2007) which examined ways in which access was gained to information relating to health and social care provision for adults with physical impairments highlighted ways in which access to information could, and needed to, improve. Likewise, analysed study data demonstrated how a lack of access to current and relevant information about available local mental health services had been a major barrier to many women's efforts to access their required support, with the majority of women emphasising the vital role of information in enabling people to access services appropriate to meeting their needs. Where information was available, frustration was consistently voiced at the use of language or jargon which was not always understood, alongside a failure to clearly outline what individual services or facilities provided their eligibility criteria and accessibility for disabled people. For Helen, unsuccessful attempts to identify localised services had led her to believe that no statutory sector provision existed within her home locality and subsequently focused her searches elsewhere:

> Back in the late eighties when I was looking for help with my anxiety and depression I couldn't find anything yet thought I was looking in all the right places – doctor's surgery, libraries, etc. and in the end [I] just thought nothing existed. I approached private agencies that advertised their services in telephone directories but their charges were way beyond what I could afford then. After what seemed like ages a social worker referred me to a mental health day centre where I found all sorts of information on posters, leaflets and from other people there about services which I could potentially access … it was as if they didn't want to publicise the services too much for fear of the demand becoming too great.
>
> Helen (age 41, congenital impairment)

A similar view was shared by two women who perceived service information to be increasingly rationed whilst cuts to services were taking place at a time when demand for mental health services was growing. Lisa recalled her frustration in seeking information about services which may assist in addressing her mental distress:

> When I was going through a low patch I didn't particularly want to speak to my GP, partly due to past experiences but was just looking for maybe a support group or somewhere you could go and chat to others going through the stuff you were but there seemed to be very little available. Eventually I went to my doctor and got referred to a psychiatric nurse and when she visited well suddenly you were given all this information about local services … it was as if you have to wait until you're bad enough to need professional help before you get access to this sort of information but if I'd known about the services earlier I might have not suffered in the way I did.
>
> Lisa (age 45, congenital impairment)

However, women who had sought information about mental health services in more recent years commented on an increasing use of information technology and how service information, in particular those provided through the statutory sector, had been obtained through internet searching. Whilst this development was broadly welcomed, caution was also expressed about an over-reliance on information technology given that access to the internet either at home or in public buildings such as libraries should neither be assumed to be universally accessible, nor that all individuals will have the required knowledge to locate the information they were seeking. Two women commented on how the voluntary sector support groups they regularly attended survived on shoestring budgets and consciously did not publicise their services widely due to an inability to cater for large numbers of people resulting from gradual declines in their subsidised funding. Additionally, for some women the issue of not feeling motivated to seek support or information when experiencing mental distress needed to be recognised, with a shared belief in it being a part of the mental health workers role to inform those with whom they work about locally available services which may potentially offer benefit.

Waiting for Services

The well-documented increasing demands being placed on community and in-patient mental health services UK-wide in the early twenty-first century, and the work pressures on the professionals working within them, were recognised group-wide. However, for the large majority of women, waiting times to gain access to a service or a professional were strongly felt to have been excessive with many believing that delays in referrals to appropriate agencies being actioned had exacerbated their distress.

Having been referred to statutory mental health agencies for treatment and/or support, typically by a GP, lengthy waits for an initial assessment of need by a mental health professional were shown to have been commonplace; whilst women referred to community mental health teams for an assessment typically by community psychiatric nurses experienced waiting times of between six weeks to three months, waiting times of approximately a year for an initial assessment by a local health trust-based clinical psychologist were reported by five women. Similarly, waiting times of approximately eight months to see a psychologist were considered unacceptable by three women given the severity of the mental distress they perceived themselves to be experiencing, the prolonged waiting then having exacerbated their upset and anxiety. With similar sentiments echoed by fellow participants, Claire described her frustration:

> When the GP suggested it may help to talk to a psychologist I was ok with that … having talked to my GP a few times it was clear he wasn't really listening though to be fair I know their time is limited. But when I got a letter telling me the waiting time for assessment was 12 months I could hardly believe it as I needed help now … Then I found out it would likely be another couple of months before the therapy process really began, it was crazy. I knew my distress needed help now and in the end a couple of weeks later I ended up in hospital due to being so unwell.
>
> Claire (age 39, acquired spinal illness)

Endeavours to access counselling through organisations affiliated to their respective impairments (Multiple Sclerosis Society and The Stroke Association) were described by two women, with each organisation promoting the specialist counselling and emotional support they offered to people living with those conditions. Both women hoped that the respective organisations would provide them with counselling support within a reasonable waiting time however, the reality had been waiting times on a par with statutory sector provision due to the organisations employing a small number of counsellors who covered large geographical areas. Furthermore, they were only able to offer a maximum of four counselling sessions per individual resulting from budget cuts by local authorities.

The Role of the General Practitioner

For 10 women, their GPs had been the initial point of contact when seeking mental health support, and analysed data affirmed women's perception of the vital role played by GPs in determining whether or not services were accessed, in particular with regard to statutory sector provision. Likewise, a good pre-existing relationship between the woman and her GP alongside a good knowledge of her specific circumstances were considered key to accessing appropriate service provision with Jackie having firmly believing that her long-term relationship with her GP, combined with being familiar with her medical history, had been instrumental in her request for counselling being dealt with promptly. Of the 12 women, only three rated the support provided by their GP within the context of their experiences of mental distress as 'good' or 'very good', both in terms of providing initial support and in subsequently making referrals to the appropriate agencies as was deemed necessary.

Amongst the nine women who rated their GP's response as 'poor' or 'mediocre' there existed a consensus that their actions had been both inadequate and not in line with the support being sought. Voicing sentiments that were mirrored by several women, Philippa recalled her GP's failure to grasp the depth of her distress:

> Although I was quite depressed I put off going to my GP for a while as from past experiences I'd often felt he didn't take my depression seriously and just thought it was because of my disability that I was a bit down. But as things got worse I really needed help ... we asked for a home visit which was refused so someone went to the surgery and told them how bad I was ... basically hysterical ... within half an hour a doctor turned up and three hours later a psychiatrist arrived but to this day I know the GP only came because family made a fuss and the home visit request shouldn't have ever been questioned ... it was something asked for out of desperation.
>
> Philippa (age 36, congenital impairment)

Consistently demonstrated by the data was how the habitual response of a GP to a woman self-presenting and expressing feelings of low mood had been to prescribe anti-depressant medication. Several women recalled scenarios in which their GP had listened for a short while before prescribing anti-depressants and recommending an appointment one month later if there had been no improvements in their symptoms. Whilst the work and time pressures GPs routinely worked under were widely recognised, the majority of women felt anti-depressants and/or medications used to treat symptoms of mental or psychological distress were prescribed too readily and that lengthier dialogue between GP and patient (women and men) was needed concerning their willingness or otherwise to take any suggested medications. Furthermore, a belief that GPs had often been slow to refer on to mental health services was voiced by several women who were acutely aware that drug medication in isolation was likely to provide limited benefits. Similarly, women dissatisfied with the support provided by their GP further believed that their delaying making referrals to mental health agencies had in part been a consequence of the increasing demands over recent years on mental health services with GPs perceived by some women to be acting as gatekeepers to services.

Mental Health Support within Rehabilitation

Difficulties in accessing mental health support have been written about by a small number of women with acquired impairments (Morris 1989, Keith 1996, Smith 2003). After acquiring her spinal injury, Morris described how her rehabilitation programme had focused almost entirely on improving functional ability and with no opportunity provided to talk about any psychological and emotional needs (Morris 1989). Morris's experiences were mirrored by three women with acquired impairments within my study, each of whom had endured long stays on spinal injury rehabilitation wards. Over recent years, the argued need for counselling to be part of the process of rehabilitation has been commented upon (Etherington 2002, Griffiths 2002, Spinal Cord Injury Association 2005), and like Morris, Jackie and Claire recalled rehabilitation programmes which, in the late 1970s, had focused on functional recovery, bladder control and regaining independence. Conversely, psychological needs had overwhelmingly been ignored by medical and nursing staff alike, with emotional support having been provided almost solely by fellow patients:

> The emotional support that patients gave each other was something I valued highly as to varying degrees we were going through the same things and had similar feelings even though I was much younger than most of the other patients. I don't mean disrespect to people who have gone through training and got qualifications but I think in situations like mine there can be no substitution for personal experience and unless you have been through something like this yourself you can't begin to truly understand what it's like.
>
> Jackie (age 45, acquired spinal cord injury)

Currently attending annual check-up reviews within the same Spinal Injuries Unit where she was treated in the immediate months post-injury, Jackie however applauded the steadily increased focus on a multi-disciplinary approach which she had increasingly observed over the last decade. As a result of the shift in focus, psychological and emotional issues were now being routinely considered alongside any physical health issues:

> The spinal injuries unit now is unrecognisable to what it was then … I go once a year for an overall check-up and for many years it just used to focus entirely on all the physical stuff to do with spinal injuries but for the past seven or eight years it's been a much wider approach and among other people you get to see a psychologist … they don't offer ongoing help but if there are concerns they will follow them through with their counterparts in your home area … it's been a big change and a welcome one.
>
> Jackie (age 45, acquired spinal cord injury)

Jackie's positive experience contrasted however with that of Judith who, following a stroke in 2008 had found there to be no psychological support available either during her prolonged stay on a rehabilitation unit or following her discharge:

> When I had my stroke it was very sudden and after the initial blur things hit me hard … I was anxious about if I'd walk again or get back to work, paying the rent, looking after my home, all sorts of things as overnight it all changed.

> Nobody seemed able to answer my questions it was always 'wait and see' and I got very down especially when my progress was so slow. Family asked if I could talk to a counsellor or someone but was told there wasn't anyone at that time and that it was normal to feel like that after a stroke. By the time I went home none of my psychological stuff had really been considered and I was left to sort all that pretty much myself.
>
> Judith (age 61, acquired paralysis following stroke)

The contrasting experiences of two women within the same time era possibly suggests geographical variation in provision and that arguably there remains significant progress to be made in meeting any psychological health needs of women with acquired impairments. Findings from a study conducted by The Stroke Association (The Stroke Association 2013) which examined the psychological impact for individuals who had suffered a stroke found that too many stroke survivors (and their families) had felt abandoned after leaving hospital and felt they had been left without the support they required to cope with the emotional impact of stroke. In emphasising how the emotional effects of stroke could be as devastating as the physical effects, the study called for greater recognition by health and social care professionals of the emotional impact of suffering a stroke, claiming that increased recognition would hopefully assist people in receiving a comprehensive assessment of their needs, and subsequently be provided with appropriate support without which could arguably impact on and delay the recovery process. Of the 2,711 people interviewed across the UK, over half (59 per cent) reported feeling depressed in the months following their stroke, 67 per cent had experienced anxiety considered to be as a direct result of their stroke, 43 per cent had experienced anger and 73 per cent a lack of confidence. Additionally, 53 per cent had experienced difficulties in their relationship with their spouse or partner, with three of those 10 people revealing how the impact of their stroke had either led to the break-up of their relationship or, were considering a break up due to the strain placed on the relationship resulting from the stroke. Whilst 42 per cent of participants had felt abandoned by health and social care professionals, an overwhelming 79 per cent had received no information or practical advice to help them cope with the emotional impact of stroke (The Stroke Association 2013). Such findings were likely to have been considered by the Stroke Association to be disappointing given their close resemblance to the views expressed by stroke survivors in a similar study which the organisation undertook seven years previously (Stroke Association 2006) and with similar findings highlighted within my own research (Smith 2003, 2010). Collectively, such findings present an unfavourable and disappointing indicator of a continuing failure to provide adequate psychological support to individuals who become physically impaired as a result of stroke (or other sudden onset traumas or conditions) and who, in the months following onset of impairment, experience mental distress.

Using Mental Health Services

In addition to the barriers and/or difficulties encountered when accessing mental health services, the study findings showed women to have encountered a range of barriers and/or difficulties when using services and receiving mental health support, and which will be considered below.

Awareness and Understanding of Impairment and Disability

Firstly, clearly evidenced by the research findings was that poor experiences of using mental health services had occurred repeatedly where the mental health professional with whom the women had worked was perceived as having a limited understanding and/or awareness of disability and impairment, with two thirds of women considering the support and/or treatment they had received from a spectrum of health and social care professionals to have been inappropriate to their needs as disabled women. Further, the majority of women considered their worker, for the most part had perceived their client to be a 'tragic' person living with a terrible 'illness', being particularly prevalent for women with acquired impairments and reinforced further where an impairment had been acquired at a young age and/or suddenly. Mixed experiences of receiving support were additionally attributed by two women to being asked to talk within their counselling sessions about areas of their lives which women had felt to be irrelevant to the mental distress they were experiencing and exacerbated by the professionals perceived inability to listen to the words the woman was saying, thus creating a barrier to forging an effective working relationship. By focusing on her dependency on others for help with daily living as being a part explanation for her mental distress, Philippa considered her CPN's approach had been unhelpful:

> The CPN always wanted to talk about how she could understand my breakdown because of my daily life and always needing help from others. It took ages for her to accept that my breakdown was totally unrelated as I'd needed help for many years … it was just part of my everyday life. Why she fixated on it I don't know but she'd had no previous experience of working with someone in a wheelchair and eventually admitted it was all new to her.
>
> Philippa (age 36, congenital impairment)

In contrast to reported negative experiences of using mental health services, positive experiences were seen to have occurred in instances where the mental health or allied professional was perceived as having a good awareness and understanding of impairment and disability in addition to being knowledgeable about the social model of disability and its principles (Kennedy 2007). Furthermore, these professionals had listened to the women's thoughts around possible contributory factors to their experiences of mental distress and had been open to exploring these within their working relationship.

Whilst several women affirmed a personal belief in counselling as an effective form of treatment for their mental distress, the need for individuals to be prepared to commit to the therapy process even though potentially it may be difficult and/or painful was emphasised. Many women described undergoing counselling as a difficult process because of the issues they had been required to open up and talk about, but in persevering the process had for some been considered worthwhile with noticeable improvement in their mental and psychological health reported by the end of the counselling process. Of the 10 women who underwent counselling on one or more occasions, six believed the process had enabled them to recognise personal strengths which prior to entering into counselling they had been unaware they possessed with their self-esteem and confidence having also improved. Positive experiences were also reported by four women who considered that counselling had enabled them to develop coping mechanisms in addition to having provided them with the confidence that if further episodes of mental distress were experienced in future, that they would feel able to work through their mental health issues either independently or with the support of family and friends.

Length of Contact with Mental Health Services

Further highlighted as a negative element of the experiences of several women was that when a mental health service or professional had been accessed, that the number of therapy or contact sessions allocated to them, and the time span over which they took place had been considered insufficient for their needs. Group-wide, women acknowledged the continuous pressures and demands placed upon statutory and non-statutory sector services and that open ended contact for any individual, except in the most exceptional circumstances was unlikely to be feasible or affordable. However, women highlighted the need for professionals to give greater consideration to the possibility of disabled clients having specific needs in addition to offering increased flexibility in the number of counselling sessions offered, determined both by the nature of the individual's mental health issues and the acuteness of the distress being experienced.

Helen described her repeated frustrations when receiving NHS counselling;

> The introductions, making sure I was comfortable sitting where I was in my wheelchair, it all took time given my speech difficulties and often there didn't seem much time left. It got to be frustrating as I'd invested so much energy just in getting ready and then getting there to seemingly not achieve a great deal yet left knowing it would be another three weeks before your next appointment.
>
> Helen (age 41, congenital impairment)

A small number of women expressed satisfaction with receiving counselling or another form of mental health support over a set time frame, with the purpose of addressing specific issues and concluding involvement when the agreed goals set between the professional and themselves had been achieved. Conversely, women living with life limiting or progressive impairments expressed a wish for longer term or open ended access to a named worker, which for Elisabeth would have provided a safety net at times of need;

> My condition is life limiting and over time my capabilities have declined … as major declines happen these can get me down mentally and they may be two weeks apart or two years you just don't know but going through them I might feel a need to talk to someone but each time you have to get re referred and wait all over again … . most times it's someone different to the person before so they don't know you at all and it's back to square one and really frustrating. It would be great if I just had a named person as it's not to say you'd be calling them all the time but just at times of need you would know the support was there …
>
> Elisabeth (age 62, congenital impairment)

Additionally, analysed data evidenced the importance that women attached to having the opportunity to work with the same professional for the duration of the time they were receiving mental health support, regardless of the length of contact, with a consistency of worker perceived to be a key element in providing optimum opportunity to develop a good working relationship. Where a change of worker had occurred due to sickness absence or a change of employment, a sense of disruption and frustration had been experienced in particular by women who had had frequent and/or longer term contact with a mental health service, with contrasting experiences described by Lisa:

> The first time I was allocated to a community mental health nurse it worked out ok as we got on well and contact was regular and scheduled but the second time a few years later the nurse was constantly off sick which I know can't always be helped but it was detrimental and really impacted on my experience of that service. Eventually they allocated someone else who worked in a totally different way and it was hard to adjust … for me I think consistency of worker really affects your experiences of using services as I've experienced the good and the bad.
>
> Lisa (age 45, congenital impairment)

In-patient Care

As the sole participant with experience of in-patient psychiatric care during the 1980s and 1990s, Claire's experiences were consistently rated as poor at a number of levels with a recurrent theme of medical and nursing staff who were perceived as lacking a basic awareness and/or understanding of issues around impairment and disability, and whom with few exceptions, assumed her acute mental distress to have been an inevitable response to her life experiences during adolescence. A first admission to an adolescents unit for young people with mental health issues in the late 1980s had resulted from significant weight loss, with the focus of the eight month stay having been on weight gain but with minimal opportunity for Claire to explore with ward professionals the underlying reasons for her eating distress. Upon reaching her target weight Claire was discharged home with little aftercare and subsequently was twice readmitted having lost the weight gained during her admission.

With no previous experience of treating a wheelchair-user patient, nursing staffs understanding of Claire's mobility and personal care needs had been limited and throughout her lengthy admission Claire had felt trapped in an environment where she did not belong:

> The girls' part of the ward was almost full of girls with anorexia ... many would have to sit alongside staff at mealtimes to ensure they ate their meals but then would return to their bed spaces and exercise so as to burn off calories ... this was a different world to mine and I never knew this stuff happened. I just thought I was there to get well again as a body weight of just over 5 stone aged 19 was supposedly dangerously low ... I never knew they'd given me a diagnosis of anorexia nervosa until a couple of months into the admission and it was a real shock ... I wasn't like these girls who would pinch their bodies before going to bed to see if there were any areas of fat on their bodies and everything was alien to me.
>
> Claire (age 39, acquired spinal illness)

Further admissions during the 1990s had disappointingly for Claire remained characterised by environments that were not wheelchair accessible despite the units being newly built, with an absence of call buzzers in bedrooms or bathrooms and a lack of adjustable beds, pressure relieving mattresses or grab rails further reinforcing the unsuitability of the environment for meeting her nursing or physical care needs. A lack of suitable aids and adaptations had consequently resulted in an increased level of dependency on others for help with personal care and daily living tasks that had not always been forthcoming, with Claire describing fellow patients as having a better understanding of her mobility requirements than nursing staff and had willingly provided any practical help she had required. Furthermore, Claire recalled mental health trained nurses focusing entirely on her mental state with only a small minority having been prepared to listen to, and learn about her physical condition and its potential to impact on mental well-being from her perspective;

> My condition can mean I have days when I'm in a lot of pain which over time does bring me down but if I asked for painkillers in the afternoon they would say well why do you want them now they aren't due until tonight and over the weeks it really got me down ... having to justify why you needed something and being a battle to get the pain relief you needed. I was determined to try and educate them as the level of ignorance and lack of awareness astounded me but it was tough.
>
> Claire (age 39, acquired spinal illness)

Following a two-month admission, at which point medical staff accepted Claire's view of the ward environment being neither suitable for her mental or physical health needs, Claire was subsequently discharged with little improvement in her mental health. Negative experiences of in-patient psychiatric care (with the exception of one admission to a specialist neuro-psychiatric unit (which will be discussed in Chapter 5) had left Claire with a pessimistic view of the availability of appropriate in-patient psychiatric care for disabled women (and men) who experience acute mental distress in the UK, and reaffirming a key finding of Morris's study (2004) which highlighted the stark polarisation of service provision for mental health service users and those for individuals with physical impairments.

In summarising her in-patient experiences, Claire spoke with pride of having no weight loss related admissions for over a decade in addition to having no involvement with community mental health services for nine years. Believing her mental health to have steadily improved over the last decade, Claire's largely negative experiences of in-patient care had ultimately led to a self-affirmation that she would never agree to a voluntary in-patient admission within an acute psychiatric ward environment during her lifetime unless some major changes at both a practical and organisational level were made. The changes that Claire and other women considered were needed will be examined in Chapter 5.

Non-statutory Provision

Local Support Groups

In contrast to the women's mixed experiences of using statutory mental health services, experiences of using non-statutory services were shown by the data to have been mostly positive and as having more beneficial outcomes. The availability of geographically local support groups had been appreciated by four women, both for their referral processes having been overall less bureaucratic and protracted than their statutory counterparts, and for the opportunities they provided to meet informally and share experiences with others who were experiencing difficulties similar to their own. Whilst having initially felt reluctant to share personal thoughts with people unknown to them (and who with few exceptions were able-bodied), by listening to, and identifying with other people's experiences (albeit it by virtue of their impairment their experiences having to some degree differed), women had gradually felt more at ease and able to contribute to group discussions. Whilst Helen's speech impairment had affected her ability to contribute to group discussions, listening to others enabled her to recognise that others were experiencing feelings and thoughts akin to her own which had assisted in alleviating personal feelings of being 'abnormal':

> When I got to know about the depression support group I wasn't initially keen but my CPN said I was always saying that nobody knew what I was going through

> so to go along if only to see that there were others experiencing difficulties that may not be exactly the same but likely having similar feelings and actually she was right. Because of my speech I was quite self-conscious of speaking up but I found just listening to others helpful … it made me realise that I wasn't on my own with these thoughts and in a way it helped me to stop feeling sorry for myself all the while though I know that was part of the depression also.
>
> Helen (age 41, congenital impairment)

Similarly, a local stroke support group which enabled social contact with others had dually provided for Judith an opportunity to meet with other stroke survivors whom she perceived to have a mutual understanding of the psychological difficulties she was experiencing:

> Although the support group doesn't promote itself as a psychological, emotional support group it does so almost without trying … there's always rumours about the group closing due to a lack of funding which is always hanging over you and if the group were to fold I'd feel the loss massively. The powers that be should be providing more groups like this and not less.
>
> Judith (age 61, acquired paralysis following stroke)

Lisa, likewise echoed the mutual support she gleaned from members of an online forum set up by individuals living with the same rare genetic condition as her own:

> As my condition is quite rare it would be difficult to have local support groups and to have just a few would mean lots of travelling so the online forum was a great idea and the internet has enabled us to do that … we can leave comments at any time or have set times when people log in and have a group chat using the webcam and it works really well … I feel much less isolated and it's good to have the opportunity to chat with others who understand what I'm going through and we support each other. The fact it can be accessed from home is a bonus as a classic symptom of the condition is fatigue so having to travel to get to a group would likely mean using valuable energy. I'm proud that we set it up ourselves as there was no provision like that within the statutory services.
>
> Lisa (age 45, congenital impairment)

However, whilst advocated by some, not all women were keen on seeking psychological support through local support groups. Having attended a support group for people with eating distress, Claire had found some aspects of the available support to be beneficial. However, as the only person with impaired mobility, there were elements of the able-bodied attendees eating patterns and behaviours that she had felt unable to identify with – for example, rigorous exercise after eating – and thus had found attending the group produced limited benefits. Likewise, Philippa spoke of having been encouraged by her mental health nurse to attend a support group for people suffering from depression but had found the experience of attending to be disappointing and had provided little of benefit to improve her mental health:

> I wasn't keen on going along to the group but the community nurse kept saying I might find it helpful so really to satisfy her I went along a few times and it was quite well-attended and there were a few disabled people there so whereas I thought I'd be really self-conscious that wasn't a problem … but everyone spoke about how bad their depression was almost as if to out-do each other and if anyone suggested something that may help it would be met with a negative response and I didn't found it helped in any way. I'm sure they work for some people and may well depend on who is there but for me it wasn't a positive experience.
>
> Philippa (age 36, congenital impairment)

The availability of local support groups and their considered benefits or otherwise will be examined further in Chapter 5 which will discuss the practical and organisational changes which women considered were needed in seeking to provide in the years ahead mental health services which meet comprehensively, appropriately and effectively the needs of disabled women who experience mental distress.

The Samaritans

The vital role played by the Samaritans organisation when suffering from acute mental distress was emphasised by each of the seven women who had used the telephone service on one or more occasions. The Samaritans' 24-hour, 365-days-a-year availability had provided a great source of reassurance whilst the confidential telephone helplines were valued for eliminating any concerns around physical accessibility. The absence of time constraints placed on phone calls were likewise welcomed, especially by women who had been anxious about making contact but had been put at ease by the call handlers' sensitive approach to listening and questioning, and consequently had felt able to talk about the distress they were experiencing. However, the limitations of telephone contact for individuals with communication impairments were recognised and whilst email communication was now offered by the Samaritans (for those with access to the internet), a preference for a listening ear on the end of a phone had been favoured by most women, in particular when experiencing acute distress. As a user of Samaritans telephone help lines over many years, Claire described her experience:

> For me the Samaritans has been an absolute lifeline at times … on one occasion it was literally a call I made when on the verge of taking an overdose that stopped me in my tracks and in my mind I know I would have gone through with it … I was so distressed. Often of course things seem worse in the middle of the night and that's when the Samaritans have been there when other services haven't …

> Now of course even local authorities have their crisis teams which offer phone access but for me it was the confidentiality, the sensitivity and the non-judgmental approach the Samaritans offered which was massive when I was desperately distressed at three in the morning and could see no reason to carry on.
>
> Claire (age 39, acquired spinal illness)

Privately Funded Services

Whilst a minority of women considered their mental health issues had been satisfactorily addressed when their involvement with their worker or service had concluded, others had felt, to varying degrees that their mental health issues had not been sufficiently addressed and subsequently sought privately funded support. However, the high costs of private counselling meant it had only been affordable to three women (of whom two for only a short period of time) with both having found a change of counsellor to be disruptive and not beneficial due to their new workers adopting different approaches in their work to what they had become familiar with. Additionally, both women highlighted the lengthy time and energy invested in identifying a private counsellor whose work location met their mobility requirements. Concern was similarly expressed that the counselling had needed to be self-funded and the costs of which had meant sacrifices needing to be made in other areas of their lives, and group-wide women believed that where a need for counselling or another form of mental health support had been identified, that it should be available through statutory or non-statutory services and without costs being incurred by any individual.

Through her direct payments funding (via which Helen received a monthly payment from her local authority based on an assessment of her care needs to arrange her own care package), Helen had considered herself fortunate to be able to finance private counselling as part of a comprehensive care package which likewise had provided her with a level of control over the support she received. Whilst being aware of a need to not become dependent on counselling, and to continue only whilst there was a real need, private counselling with a male counsellor with whom Helen had established a good rapport was believed to have assisted in maintaining her positive mental well-being, thus contrasting with her previously experienced anxieties when the counselling process with NHS counsellors was nearing completion.

Conclusions

Within this chapter any barriers that had been encountered in gaining access to mental health services and women's subsequent experiences of using services have been examined. In endeavouring to gain access to services, the chapter has highlighted how for the majority of women accessing mental health support had not been an easy process with similar barriers to access highlighted across the sample group, specifically within the statutory sector, whilst inaccessible service locations had been particularly problematic for women seeking support prior to the introduction of anti-discrimination legislation. Improved support from GPs, who for most women had been the first point of contact following the onset of mental distress, and a wider availability of current information about mental health services were stressed as being vital in enabling the process of accessing appropriate support to commence in earnest.

Experiences of using mental health services and their effectiveness in addressing women's mental distress was shown for most women to have been affected by a perceived lack of awareness and understanding around disability and impairment amongst the professionals with whom women had worked. Whilst varying levels of dissatisfaction were expressed concerning the timescales women were offered with a mental health professional or service and negative aspects of in-patient care were highlighted by the one participant who had experienced in-patient psychiatric care within various locations, more positive experiences of receiving support from services in the non-statutory sector such as the Samaritans were emphasised. Based on women's experiences of both accessing and using mental health services, a number of both organisational and practical changes were identified which women believed if applied, would improve both service provision and increased positive reporting of using mental health services and subsequently resulting in improved mental health and well-being. These changes will be examined in detail within Chapter 5.

Chapter 3
Counselling, Disabled People and Loss

Introduction

Within the existing body of literature that is concerned with counselling and physical impairment there exists an overall agreement that historically as a client group, disabled people have not been well served by counsellors or allied professionals who provide counselling as part of their work role with disabled people. A review commissioned by the Joseph Rowntree Foundation in the early 1990s which examined both the need for, and the availability of counselling for disabled people, highlighted mainstream counsellors' lack of experience of working with disabled clients and their minimal understanding of the likely issues raised by living with a physical impairment. Study participants (in particular those with acquired impairments) considered that access to counselling and emotional support would have been beneficial in the immediate months following onset of their impairment with the review concluding that disabled people needed a counselling service which met their needs as they perceived them (Social Policy Unit 1992). This view was repeated by disabled women within Lonsdale's study (1990) who voiced a need for counselling at different stages of their lives, whilst those with acquired impairments recalled how counselling would have been welcomed in the months following onset of impairment but had seldom been offered. A small scale study which examined the mental health experiences of a small group of disabled women (Smith 2003) similarly highlighted how access to counselling provision had been particularly problematic.

Within this chapter the expansion of both UK counselling provision and counselling literature since the latter decades of the twentieth century will firstly be examined with a particular focus on the development of counselling provision aimed specifically at women. Whilst sections of the counselling literature have focused on working with women within different client groups, the potential specific needs of disabled women have been paid little attention and counsellors' perceptions of physical impairment and their possible concerns and anxieties around working with disabled clients will be considered in addition to looking at the anxieties of disabled people within the context of the counselling process. The chapter will then consider the concept of loss, and the central role of theories of loss in informing the medical model of disability has attracted wide criticism for a failure to acknowledge the repercussions of living within a society that historically has contained a set of beliefs and practices about disabled people. The disempowering nature of loss theories and alternative approaches to loss, which in recent years have been presented as providing a more accurate representation of how individuals respond to impairment, will be considered before examining women's personal views on experiences of loss.

A lack of approaches within the counselling literature that are informed by the social model of disability, and which recognise the potential for oppression within the counsellor-client relationship, combined with little or no teaching about disability as an equal opportunities issue within counselling training have resulted in stereotypes and prejudices in society about disability and impairment being neither exposed or challenged by counsellors. In responding to such criticisms, the chapter will finally consider the suggested benefits or otherwise of counselling approaches which have been advocated as being appropriate for counsellors to utilise when working with disabled clients who require counselling support.

Defining Counselling

In recent decades, arguably the most outstanding feature of the development and provision of counselling in the UK as a form of treatment or psychological support has been its expansion alongside an emerging body of literature which has examined counselling processes when working with a wide range of client groups or circumstances such as counselling work with children, relationship or bereavement counselling (Lago 2007, Dryden and Mytton 1999). In addition, since the early 1990s the number of trained counsellors within the UK has increased significantly with a number of factors identified as having contributed to this growth (McLeod 1998).

Until the 1980s caring and 'people' professions such as nursing, teaching and social work had provided a quasi-counselling role, after which time their roles began to be financially and managerially squeezed resulting in some members of such professions seeking training as counsellors and creating specialist counselling roles within their organisations as a way of maintaining direct contact with their clients. The areas of overlap between counselling and other forms of help such as social work, community nursing and even everyday friendship were highlighted by Feltham and Dryden (1993) as was the existence of contrasting definitions and interpretations arising from the process by which counselling had developed. The literature contains a range of definitions of counselling with its variety demonstrating the different meanings that it has for different people. For McLeod counselling is:

> an activity that has emerged within Western society in the twentieth century as a means of providing and maintaining individualism and the sense of a person as an autonomous self.
>
> McLeod 1998: 3

The British Association of Counselling and Psychotherapy place an emphasis on exploration and understanding rather than action and define counselling as:

> an opportunity for the client to work towards living in a way that he/she experiences as being more satisfying and resourceful.
>
> BACP 1998

During the twentieth century, counselling evolved and changed rapidly and itself became contained within a variety of different themes, emphases, practices and schools of thought (McLeod 1998). Currently in the early twenty-first century three core approaches to counselling are widely recognised, namely the *psycho-dynamic, behavioural* and *humanistic* approaches, with each representing fundamentally different ways of viewing human beings and their emotional and behavioural problems. Whilst counsellors working within a psycho-dynamic approach focus primarily on insight, those adopting a humanistic approach within their work with clients aim to promote self-acceptance and personal freedom whilst cognitive behavioural therapists are mainly concerned with the management and control of behaviour. Likewise, underlying the diversity of theoretical models there exists within counselling literature a variety of ideas expressed about the aims of counselling with McLeod amongst others suggesting that these aims relate implicitly or explicitly to insight, self-awareness and empowerment (McLeod 1998).

Over recent decades, additionally witnessed has been a significant growth in the diversity of counselling practice available with counselling in the early twenty-first century now being delivered in a variety of ways, for example, through one to one contact, group or family counselling, telephone counselling, self-help manuals or peer counselling. Furthermore, the technological advances of recent years have led to an increased availability of online counselling via written dialogue or verbal conversation using a webcam facility. In addition, the number of people who have turned to counselling in recent decades to help resolve personal difficulties in their lives has increased including disabled women (and men) who are seeking therapeutic support which meets their perceived needs and which may be related among other factors to stress, relationship problems or issues associated with impairment or disability.

Women and Counselling

A number of contributors to the counselling literature over recent years have claimed that organisations which provide counselling services to women have had a significant impact both on the current understanding of women's psychology and on the issues that women explore in counselling, with the development of counselling within women's organisations having been influenced by many factors (Perry 1993, Boswell and Poland 2003). In particular, a wish to respond to the 'whole woman' and efforts to move away from relating to the woman as someone defined only in relation to others, so valuing a woman's essentially in her own right have been a primary concern (Nairn and Smith 1986, Miles 1988, Busfield 1992, 1996, Chaplin 1999, Kohen 2000).

A second significant strand since the latter decades of the twentieth century has been the establishment of women's self-help groups such as Women's Aid, community-based counselling services within Family Support Units and Anorexic Aid, all of which arose in response to a perceived lack of counselling provision within the statutory sector. The growth of the women's self-help movement across the UK, working with the belief that support is most effectively provided by women who have shared similar experiences, together with women's therapy centres have been far reaching with their projects having provided valuable examples of women working effectively with each other in ways which appreciate and value women's strengths and characteristics. Likewise, within such settings women's views are listened to in earnest whilst their needs and circumstances are effectively acknowledged and addressed within the counselling process.

In contrast to white, male, euro-centric models of counselling in which the emphasis has traditionally been on getting down to business straight away (Walker 1990), the importance of workers within women's organisations consciously providing a warm and welcoming counselling environment in which women are put at ease has also been well documented within the counselling literature (McLeod 1994, Chaplin 1999, Kohen 2000). Further highlighted has been how women's ability to access and/or make optimum use of mental health/counselling services may be vitally determined by their geographical location being within a reasonable travelling distance from a home (or other) location so that other factors of women's lives are not significantly compromised, for example, their possible role as carers for family members or others, or for some combining with paid work (Barnes, Davis et al. 2002). Within the research, four women highlighted a mental health services location as having been a concern, particularly so where the location was not well served by accessible public transport which thus necessitated the additional costs of taxi transport. Similarly, participants within Jack's study which examined the counselling experiences of a group of disabled people from their own perspectives further emphasised the need for service locations to provide both disabled parking and toilet facilities (Jack 2009).

In examining the development of counselling models for use when working with women, feminist counselling and therapy aimed primarily to make the counselling process both accessible and comprehensible with a simultaneous commitment to an egalitarian relationship rather than one embedded in hierarchical mode (Walker 1992). In addition, encouraging women to trust themselves and to become more assertive, endeavouring to enable women to acknowledge and express anger and women's voices being neither invalidated nor repressed were all highlighted by McLeod (1994) as central themes within feminist therapy. Informed by a *psychotherapeutic approach*, feminist therapy has historically located the primary influences on emotion development as lying in the nature of maternal infant relations in infancy with formative effects on the impact of women's unconscious state which, have in turn inhibited conscious thoughts and actions. In contrast, the focus of feminist therapy informed by *humanistic* or *person-centred* counselling has been on how individual women have within themselves the resources for meeting their emotional needs but that their expression has been inhibited by the hostile nature of current interpersonal and social relations (McLeod 1998). The growth of feminist therapy in the later decades of the twentieth century, according to Walker (1992) resulted in an increased awareness of the impact of gender within the therapeutic process whilst also marking a radical movement away from psychological and mental health services which historically had great difficulties in understanding issues basic to women.

Within a study which examined the experiences of a group of women who underwent feminist therapy (McLeod 1994), women believed their emotional needs had had been considered to be important and that their experiences of therapy had created both a greater sense of self-worth and overall happiness. The counsellors with whom women worked were reported to have displayed a genuine concern for their welfare, with changes in the women's emotional state having represented a massive achievement set against the scale of their previous distress and the input of prior relationships and treatment. However, despite its egalitarian intent, a number of shortcomings within the feminist therapy approach have been commented upon which critics believe may potentially result in an inability to resolve the inequalities implicated in women's mental distress. For example, despite its self-help ethos, the counsellor–client relationship has been considered to be intrinsically hierarchical, therefore giving rise to a danger that the woman in therapy may defer to the counsellor's view of the nature of their problem as opposed to being able to express these without inhibition and thereby gaining some true resolution of them (McLeod 1994). Further, critics have argued that women's emotional needs may be subordinated by their differential experiences as women from ethnic minorities, lesbian women etc. which suggests that feminist therapy cannot be assumed to take account of the diversity of women's experiences for example, those of disabled women with the process of feminist counselling according to Dobash and Dobash (1992) arguably having the pathologising effect of defining emotional suffering as rooted in problems in the woman's personality. Therefore, feminist therapy, it is suggested should only be seen as a partial solution to the problem of securing women's emotional well-being with a comprehensive realisation requiring, according to McLeod, (1994) a more complex and extensive range of initiatives which, combined with feminist therapy tackle the unequal nature of social relations beyond gender subordination alone.

In addressing the controversial issue of whether counsellors should have personal experience of inequality in order to be able to provide counselling support, Burstow (1992) believes it possible for counsellors to respond in a way that is useful through awareness and sensitivity towards conditions of which they may lack personal experience. However, contributions from lesbian women (Perkins 1991) and black women (Birmingham Council Black Women's Unit 1995) have suggested that it is only when women organise on the basis of first-hand experiences of social dimensions *other than* gender that their significance for shaping the emotional well-being of the women themselves starts to become apparent. This topic shall be explored further within Chapter 4 where the emerging debate of recent years concerning whether disabled people should be counselled by disabled counsellors will be discussed.

Counselling and Disability

As stated within the Introduction, historically, as a client group, disabled people of both sexes have overall not been well served by counsellors, psychologists or allied health and social care professionals who provide counselling as part of their work role with disabled people. In addition, a legacy of prejudicial attitudes exists with academics within disability studies (including disabled academics) having increasingly highlighted over recent years the dire need for mental health professionals to undertake more disability-related training and for more research to be undertaken within this topic area. Thus, according to Reeve (2004), whilst some disabled people manage to find counselling services that are helpful, many others are faced with inaccessible counselling agencies that have little understanding of, or insight into, the lived experience of disability (Corker 2004). Likewise, whilst recent decades have seen the expansion of counselling literature which examines and/or suggests appropriate counselling approaches when working with individuals within a range of client groups and circumstances, for example, working with young children, survivors of sexual abuse or people who have suffered a bereavement, by comparison the body of literature concerned with counselling and disabled people remains small. This absence of literature is interesting given that increasingly within recent years counselling practice texts have addressed the diverse issues raised in relation to other areas of social inequality such as gender and age, but *not* disability. However, and encouragingly, more recently the topic area has shown small signs of attracting both interest and debate which hopefully will lead in future to a growing and varied literature within a long neglected subject area.

Counsellors' Perceptions of Physical Impairment

In a study by Parkinson (2006) which explored the attitudes of 25 trainee and practising counsellors towards disabled people, both their perception of disability in general and how counsellors felt they may approach a disabled client were examined. The study findings showed 75 per cent to have viewed impairment in terms of either a tragedy or a form of irrevocable loss, with unanimous surprise expressed when fed back to participants with none having considered themselves to be conscious of such attitudes until raised within the discussion group. Further highlighted was a general consensus that counsellors' attitudes to, and beliefs about disability and impairment should be explored in depth as part of disability equality training sessions, claiming that where DET had to date been included, that the focus had been on the individual's impairment, with its content reflecting a remit to 'treat' or 'alleviate' the impairment and to make the individual as 'normal' as possible (Parkinson 2006). In so doing, this does little to assist any attempts to remove the physical and psychological exclusion of disabled people and conversely could be seen as perpetuating the negative barriers that such services aim to remove (Beckett and Wrighton 2000).

In her writings on disability and counselling, Wilson (2003) cites the example of a disabled woman who entered into counselling with a counsellor whose initial desire had been to take control of the woman and make her physical condition 'better' but an inability to bring about a physical change in their client had created for the counsellor a sense of helplessness and frustration. Through becoming aware of and acknowledging this, Wilson believed a mismanagement of the forged relationship to have been prevented with the counsellor having additionally been provided with a glimpse into the woman's ongoing daily life experiences, thus resulting in the creation of common ground for building a fuller understanding of her client's predicament. Like other mental health and social care professionals, Wilson believes that counsellors will often experience an internal struggle between the omnipotent wish to make a difference by appearing strong and able whilst an acknowledgement of one's own limitations and frustrations are a pre-requisite for empathy and understanding, and that only by being able to let go of their fantasy of being a saviour can counsellors arrive at a more realistic perception of their role. Simultaneously, counsellors become aware that their task is neither to change nor to improve their client's physical condition, but to participate in a mutual process in which clients are assisted to develop their autonomy. In letting go of the fantasy, it is claimed that counsellors and allied professionals may find themselves confronted not only by their client's perceived helplessness and vulnerability but also their own. Thus, according to Wilson, it is the discomfort caused by close proximity to the fragility of human existence that is potentially one of the likely reasons why many counsellors have anxieties about working with disabled clients or as a specialism with their unsuccessful endeavours to locate a counsellor who specialised in working with disabled clients recalled by three women.

As a result of the lack of attention which Lago and Smith (2004) argue has historically been devoted to issues around equal opportunities within the training courses of counsellors (and potentially other health and social care professionals who may provide counselling as part of their role in working with disabled clients), Reeve considers it to be almost inevitable that non-disabled counsellors will experience some form of fear or anxiety about disability and impairment. Furthermore, as a result, attention is unlikely to be paid to their own attitudes, fears and prejudices of a conscious or unconscious nature, and which if left unnoticed could both limit the congruence and empathy of counsellors and potentially contaminate clear communication (Reeve 2000). A consideration of the need for both disability equality training and teaching around the social model of disability to be included within the training courses of counsellors (and other professionals who may provide counselling to disabled clients as part of their work role) will be examined within Chapter 5.

Furthermore, the scarcity of disabled students in the classroom may arguably result in disability 'not being present' in the room in the same way that gender, ethnicity and sexuality are likely to be. In examining the scarcity of disabled counsellors in the UK through the 1990s, Withers (1996) highlighted the experiences of a small number of disabled counsellors who for the duration of their training courses reported having to deal with reactions of pity and embarrassment both from prejudiced tutors and fellow students.

For counsellors, their anxieties may take the form of:

- Fear of disabled people as threatening others; if a non-disabled counsellor is afraid of what a disabled client represents to him or her, they may develop a subtle distant and uninvolved attitude which disabled people could experience or interpret as rejection (Wilson 2003).
- Feeling helpless and powerless that as counsellors they are unable to make their client 'better' and being able-bodied, may feel guilty for being 'well' (Parkinson 2006).
- Over-emphasising the positives; disabled people may feel a need to conform to social and cultural expectations by overcoming their impairments and counsellors may collude by responding to the positive aspects of the disabled client's experience more than to any difficulties the client may have in being disabled (Reeve 2000).

Disabled Clients: Barriers to the Counselling Relationship

Whilst counsellors may have anxieties about working with disabled clients, barriers to positive counselling relationships may also be experienced by disabled clients and whilst the value of counselling for disabled people has been endorsed by some (Griffiths and Weyman 2003, Smith 2003), others are sceptical about its value (Reeve 2000, Etherington 2002, Goodley 2010). As increasing numbers of able-bodied people have turned to counselling over recent decades, Lenny (1992) believes it to have become an important mechanism for addressing, if not resolving the paradox between the individual and society and that for some, counselling has been seen as a way of dealing with the relationship between their individual impairments and a disabling society. Additionally, evidence from some of the counselling and disability studies literature and research studies indicates that disabled people, like able-bodied people want access to counselling which meets their perceived needs (Lonsdale 1990, Reeve 2004, Smart and Smart 2006, Jack 2009).

According to Morris (2002), whilst physical impairment may on occasions be accompanied by chronic or intermittent episodes of illness or pain leading to periods of emotional distress, this is not always the case and people with physical impairments can be emotionally stressed in ways that are not associated with their impairment. Support for Morris' s view was clearly evident within the study data and the need for counsellors to move away from making assumptions about what disabled clients want or feel and to not act in a patronising or pitying way was further highlighted by Jack (2009) who examined from the personal perspectives of a small group of disabled adults their experiences of the counselling process. Likewise, Morgan Jones (2002) alerted counsellors to the dangers of falling into the 'reductionist trap' whereby the client was viewed firstly as 'disabled' and as a 'person' second and which was considered unlikely to enhance any therapeutic work between the counsellor and disabled client.

Disabled people's commonly expressed concerns relating to counselling include:

- They often have less choice than able-bodied people about where they receive counselling often due to a lack of suitable premises (though study findings indicated improvements in accessible environments within the past decade or so following implementation of the Disability Discrimination Act).
- Whilst peer counselling has been shown to be valued by some it is not available in all parts of the UK. Where offered to a disabled individual, peer counselling may not be their preferred counselling method but may be accepted due to it often having shorter waiting times than statutory sector counselling.
- For those not in employment or unable to work and therefore with less disposable income, private practice is likely to be unaffordable unless reasonable adjustments linked to specific needs and circumstances are made.
- That counsellors are not sufficiently informed about the impact of the physical and social environment for disabled people on both physical and emotional well-being (Swain, Griffiths and Heyman 2003).
- That counselling often takes place within medical or voluntary settings, both of which may reinforce the established cultural view of disability as a medical condition and disabled people as objects of charity and pity. Such settings may for some disabled people also be associated with negative experiences, for example, treatment or surgery linked to impairments which may have been experienced as painful or environments where people had unwanted diagnoses confirmed.
- That counsellors fail to give due consideration to client's capabilities, often instead emphasising their deficiencies (Shakespeare 2006).

Counselling and Loss

Where theories of loss have been examined within the social psychology and psychiatry literatures much has been written on the 'psychological problems' faced by disabled people. Commonly characterised by a medically informed personal tragedy perspective on disability (Thomas 1999) and preoccupied with issues of adjustment to, and coping with the misfortune of being disabled, personality factors were often described within the literature as being crucial to a successful or unsuccessful adjustment at the level of the individual (Woolley 1993, Hurst 2000, Morris 2002). By adopting this approach, the individual is expected to go through fixed stages of denial, anger, fear and bargaining before finally accepting the recovered stage of 'acceptance of impairment' (Reeve 2000, Sapey 2002). Likewise, such approaches predict that disabled people will grieve and negotiate their loss alongside an expectation that a period of mourning akin to that of bereavement will be gone through (Harvey 1998, Wimpenny and Costello 2011).

In an examination of the ways in which a variety of health and welfare professionals worked with disabled people, traumatised loss was defined by Berger as, among other things 'being disabled' with the phrase 'traumatic loss and disability' used in a way that combined the two and which made the assumption that to be disabled equated to having suffered a loss. An initial denial by disabled people that loss had occurred Berger (1998) suggested to be commonplace, believing that people's ability to perceive the reality of their situation was likely to be impaired, a view supported by Webb who stated that:

> grief follows inevitability from disability … all disability involves loss and if grieving is not experienced then it will be harder for other, more obvious gains to be made.
>
> Webb 1993: 202

In such circumstances disabled people may find themselves in a 'catch 22 situation' with expressions of contentment and happiness following disablement then often perceived as representing a form of denial (Lenny 1992). In particular, people with acquired impairments run the risk of being regarded as 'abnormal' and in need of psychological guidance (Oliver 1996).

The central role of theories of loss in informing the medical model of disability, and in which the 'problem' of disability is located firmly within the individual, have resulted in few writers within disability studies considering them to have merit and resulting in a number of criticisms being levelled at them. Firstly, critics have drawn attention to the failure of loss theories proponents to provide a true representation of how individuals respond to living with a physical impairment, and likewise for their lack of acknowledgement of the repercussions of living within a society that historically has contained a whole set of beliefs and practices about disability.

A dismissal within loss theories, of the possibility that a disabled person might not experience loss and an assertion that they *need* to adjust in stages to their impairment, Sapey (2004) argued indicated an ideology of superiority on the part of non-disabled people, argued by critics to be a product of the psychological imagination and constructed upon a bedrock of non-disabled people's beliefs about what it is like to experience impairment (Reeve 2000). Described by Finkelstein as 'a value judgement based on the unspoken acceptance of the standard being able-bodied normalcy' (1980: 12), critics of loss theories believe it to be able-bodied people's fear of physical impairment as being a form of death that accounted for the dominance of loss theories within the psychology of disablement throughout the mid-twentieth century, and which for many decades remained unquestioned or challenged.

In a strong rejection of traditional theories of loss, Oliver (1996) argued that many disabled people neither grieve nor mourn their impairment and that some may indeed find the experience of disability enriching. Over recent years some disabled people have begun to talk about their experience of disability as being enriching, and of how becoming disabled had opened up new and satisfying opportunities that may otherwise not have happened or been achieved (Keith 1996, Swain and French 2000, Smith 2003) whilst individuals with sufficient resources may have more time for interests and hobbies and consequently may gain a more interesting perspective on life (Vasey 1992, Greeley 1996, Smith 2003). A failure by advocates of loss theories to consider the social dimensions of disability and to assume that the sole response to impairment will be one of a person 'in loss', has attracted criticism which was further compounded by an overall failure to distinguish between any experience of loss for individuals with less severe impairments and those with life-limiting or progressive impairments. Likewise, criticism has been aimed at a failure to differentiate between any experiences of loss for individuals whose impairments were present from birth and those whose impairments are acquired.

Furthermore, critics of loss theories have argued that the *real* problems for disabled women (and men) stem from living within a disabling environment and from factors such as the potential for loss of employment or financial difficulties as opposed to the experience of physical impairment per se. Therefore, theories of loss which claimed to offer valid explanations for responses to physical impairment, Reeve (2000) believes fail to offer an explanation for the emotional distress that individuals living within a disabling environment may experience. This viewpoint was supported by Oliver (1990) who claimed that where individuals do mourn, it is their loss of independence that is being mourned and not the loss of their physical appearance or bodily functions and which was a situation that could be significantly diminished by social and environmental changes. The structural changes to the environment that have taken place since the implementation of the DDA 1995 which have resulted in improved access to public spaces and arenas for disabled people were shown by the data evidence to have impacted positively over recent years on mental well-being and is a topic which will be examined within Chapter 5.

According to Oliver, a more appropriate means of understanding the reactions of people to their change in circumstances would be to view the onset of impairment as 'a significant life event'. Whilst neither denying the likely impact of physical impairment, nor that people's experiences of life changing injuries or illness might include loss, as described by disabled women within Campling (1981), Oliver (1987) argued that such an approach calls into question the implications that established theories of loss have for people who do not conform to the stages approach. Additionally, to assume that every individual who experiences the onset of physical impairment will go through the same specified stages, or that such stages will lead to 'recovery', without attention being paid to the material and social environment was likewise considered to be inappropriate. Furthermore, by viewing the onset of impairment as 'a significant life event', Sapey (2002) suggests that it then becomes possible to include the impact of physical impairment, social responses towards physically disabled people and the meanings that individuals themselves attach to what is happening to them.

Counselling responses to disability which have been predominantly based on loss theories, have over recent years attracted wide criticism within disability studies literature and from disabled people (Thomas 1999, Olkin 1999, Watermeyer 2009) both for their disempowering nature and for reinforcing the notion that disability is an individual problem caused by impairment, as opposed to recognising society's role in both creating and maintaining disability. Predominantly, when working with disabled clients, counsellors have used approaches linked to loss with the restricted literature having subsequently arguably resulted in little meaningful discussion taking place concerning the appropriateness of loss or other counselling approaches when working with disabled clients, or indeed whether specific approaches, solely for use with disabled clients are required. In addition, an assumption within loss theories that the experience of loss is central to the life experience of disabled people has commonly been linked to the widespread societal belief that to be 'disabled' is to have a negative self-identity, with counselling thus becoming a process of helping disabled people move towards a more positive world view (Corker 2004).

In addition, the use of loss approaches within counselling, critics believe prevent counselling practice from meeting wholly client centred goals and that a focus on a positive or a negative identity within the counselling process could reinforce the medical model assumption that people *are* their impairments or experience of disability. Whilst critics have acknowledged that a struggle over identity may often be present on the agenda when disabled people seek counselling, this struggle Corker (2004) believes to not always be concerned with impairment or disability and may indeed be a consequence of a diverse range of factors, for example, continuing barriers to universally accessible public transport or the negative representation of disability in the media, though with some data evidence suggesting that a slow positive shift was currently being witnessed and which shall be discussed in later chapters. In addition, an assumption that all disabled women (and men) have a negative self-identity has been shown within recent years to be increasingly rejected by some disabled people, evidence of which was present within elements of the study data.

The diverse criticisms directed at established theories of loss have resulted in the emergence over the past decade of alternative approaches which have been presented as providing both a more realistic and accurate explanation of how individuals respond to physical impairment. Individually, the alternative approaches advocated have made a contribution to the ongoing debate within the different bodies of literature concerned with loss, disability and physical impairment and the key features of the two main proposed approaches will now be examined.

Alternative Approaches to Loss

Within the *dual process* approach, rather than going through specified stages of grief, it is suggested that people with a physical impairment will shift between a loss and a restoration orientation with either one being dominant at any one point in time. An acknowledgement of restoration orientation Sapey (2004) has claimed to be of assistance both in explaining and including the experiences of those disabled people who reject the stages approach and rather than seeking conformity to a particular model, within the dual process approach, restoration is viewed as an individual activity which is likely to draw on personal strengths and material resources. Additionally, rather than acceptance being viewed as one stage of a process, the fluctuations which may happen over a period of time and typically illustrated by anniversaries of events which may trigger an episode of grief are well-recognised within this approach. Furthermore, in representing a move away from the narrow psychologistic approach which presents grieving as a natural process, and through acknowledging the complexity of the lives that people potentially led both before and after the onset of impairment, the approach has been considered to be advantageous (Thompson 2002). Additionally, the dual process approach, Sapey (2004) claims alerts us to a complex web of socio and political factors which interact to make experiences of loss far more complex than established theories of loss would have us believe.

Secondly, the *meaning reconstruction* approach is premised on the fundamental argument that when individuals experience a profound loss, they also experience a loss of meaning and disruption of their life story; therefore within a meaning reconstruction approach the process of grieving is perceived to be one of making sense of the loss and reconstructing whatever life means, in particular those areas directly affected by loss (Thompson 2002). In reconstructing meaning after a loss, Neimeyer and Anderson (2002) identified the three important aspects as *sense making*, *benefit finding* and *identity reconstruction*. In terms of *sense making*, whilst most people will ask the question *why?* Sapey (2004) claimed that the ways in which the question is answered will vary according to a range of factors including the individual's psychological disposition, their spiritual beliefs and social support systems.

In considering *benefit finding* and *identity reconstruction*, attention is drawn to Swain and French's (2000) discussion of an affirmation of disability which claimed that disabled people have pointed to benefits they have derived from being disabled, and contrasted this with the dominant view that conceptualises disability as a personal tragedy (Sapey 2004). Additionally, attention was drawn to the way in which some disabled people had not only incorporated disability and impairment within their lives but additionally had overtly valued its inclusion within a positive identity (Swain and French 2000). Furthermore, within the meaning reconstruction approach, the need that disabled people have to establish a positive identity when aspects of their being which contributed to their overall identity have been lost is acknowledged. Where established individual models to disablement suggest that individuals will need to come to terms with change, in particular with a diminished social role and hence to accept an inferior identity, within the social model the need for the societal attitudes towards physical impairment to change is emphasised. Meaning reconstruction, according to Sapey, appears compatible with this approach through not imposing any specific mode of change but whilst simultaneously recognising that the new meanings that people reconstruct to make sense of their loss are varied (Sapey 2004).

Whilst neither the dual process nor meaning reconstruction approach deny that there can be negative consequences or experiences of living with a physical impairment and that the circumstances or situations of some individuals may be considered to be tragic, proponents of both approaches claim that an individual's response to living with, or adjusting to living with a physical impairment seldom matches the expectations of a stages approach and which will be considered below. In helping to make sense of the experiential ways in which disabled people have begun to challenge established loss theories and the notion of disability and impairment as a 'loss', Sapey considers the dual process approach to offer the clearest challenge to the 'psychological stages' theory of loss, claiming that whilst such experiences do not deny the consequences and experiences of impairment sometimes having tragic circumstances and/or causing massive upheaval to individuals' lives, they seldom match the expectations of a stages approach. Further, whilst adjusting to a sick role, Sapey (2004) argues that people do not totally put their lives on hold but take control as best as they are able and incorporate their new self into their existing life. Within the context of their personal experiences of mental distress, the research sough to examine the women's views relating to loss with data evidence displaying considerable variation in how the concept of loss was understood and where it was felt to have been experienced, in what ways. These will now be considered below.

Women and Loss: Personal Experiences

From analysed data, evident was a shared belief that where 'loss' had been experienced, and whilst similarities were evident across those experiences, ultimately any experience of loss had been unique to any individual. Furthermore, analysed data showed a group-wide agreement that the extent to which loss was experienced, (if experienced) was highly likely to be linked to the severity of the woman's impairment and the extent to which it impacted on daily life. In addition, women agreed that both the experience of loss (where it occurred), and the depth of feeling around it, were likely to depend on factors such as the woman's character and personality and that two women diagnosed with the same impairment may potentially cope with, or adapt to their 'loss' in very diverse ways. In a study which examined the daily life experiences of a group of women living with chronic physical impairments, Marris (1996) concluded that the precise nature of an individual's loss was likely to depend on factors such as the condition itself, favoured areas of work or leisure or personal desires and ambitions. Whilst Marris was unconcerned for example, that her impairment prevented her from becoming a deep sea diver or an airline pilot, there was recognition that for someone else this may represent a significant area of loss within their life.

Acquired Impairments and Loss

Amongst the six women with acquired impairments, three recalled their first experience of mental distress occurring in the initial months after onset of impairment, when the reality of their impairment and how it may affect different aspects of their future lives had been realised. Diagnosed with Multiple Sclerosis in her early thirties, Maria had experienced an array of emotions in the months following diagnosis:

> When I was diagnosed with MS I couldn't believe it … it felt like the martians had landed and that I was in a surreal place. It took me a long time to come to terms with the diagnosis and spent lots of time searching for information about it and what the implications would be for me and all of us a family.
>
> Maria (age 51, acquired neurological impairment)

For Jackie, whilst unable to pursue her dream career of veterinary medicine following a spinal injury she had proceeded to work for 20 years in full-time employment but had experienced loss when she had been unable to return to work following an acute episode of physical illness:

> Work brought a structure to my day and it made me feel normal … like I was just like other people and it was something I could do in spite of being in a wheelchair … it was good for me mentally. Work allowed me to mix with other people … it gave me a sense of being integrated into society and gave me some financial independence. When all that went it created a massive void in my life and I wasn't prepared for how it would affect me.
>
> Jackie (age 45, acquired spinal cord injury)

Jackie had also become acutely aware of her mobility limitations following the birth of her daughter and felt an acute sense of loss which was attributed to being unable to be actively involved in tasks and activities as her daughter was growing up:

> When Lucy was a baby, dad was great … he made alterations to the bath and the high chair so I could do all the normal things with her and growing up I helped with homework etc. but it was things like not being able to brush her hair, get her dressed and push her on the swings and having to watch while someone else

> did it. But that said and most importantly she got all the love in the world which doesn't need working arms and legs.
>
> Jackie (age 45, acquired spinal injury)

Whilst some women with acquired impairments considered themselves to have 'accepted' their impairments, none identified with having gone through specified 'stages' before reaching that point, with their experiences shown to be at odds with traditional loss approaches which expected individuals to grieve for their impairment. For women with acquired impairments, analysed data evidenced their processes of adjustment to have closely mirrored those outlined in the dual stages approach with 'acceptance of impairment' not perceived as a 'recovered' stage and with the majority of women recalling the process of adjusting to their impairment as having been both slow and continuous. This group of women further described 'acceptance' of their impairments to have typically shifted over a period of time with fluctuations often perceived to have resulted from external influences or factors such as anniversaries of onset of impairment. Having regained a limited level of independence during her hospital admission, Jackie believed she had 'accepted' her impairment but returning home to a partially inaccessible environment that sense of acceptance diminished having found her levels of dependency on others for help with everyday tasks had increased. Some women further recalled how, particularly in the initial years after onset, anniversaries had reinforced thoughts around their 'pre-impairment' lives and what they felt they had 'lost', thus leading them to question their 'true acceptance' but, that with the passage of time such self-questioning had diminished both in its intensity and frequency.

Congenital Impairments and Loss

For those women born with their impairments (and for whom their level of physical ability had remained relatively stable through their lives) there was a belief that whilst they had experienced 'loss' in different forms and degrees, like the women with acquired impairments, they did not identify with a stages approach to adjustment to impairment. Having developed symptoms of her genetic condition as a young child, four decades later Lisa considered herself to be '90 per cent accepting' of her impairment but that periodically she still yearned for a life that allowed her greater independence:

> Mostly I'm ok … I've found ways of doing the same everyday things as able-bodied people but just do them differently … when there's things I can't physically do I can feel a sense of loss … Like, although I was born disabled and have never known what it is to walk through sand and feel it between my toes I still wonder how it would feel. But overall I don't see it as a loss … more a sense of wondering how certain things feel … a curiosity.
>
> Lisa (age 45, congenital impairment)

For Frankie, loss had been experienced as a result of her inability to take part in school physical education activities but that her experience had been about 'feeling different' rather than a grieving process. Frankie recalled her feelings of anger and confusion when a diagnosis with which she had lived since childhood was changed in her early twenties, and was thus confronted with the reality of her impairment being a permanent feature of her life. However, whilst having gone through a process of adjusting to her physical limitations no distinct stages had been experienced. Additionally, Frankie recalled feelings of uncertainty around registering as a disabled person which were perceived to have been inextricably linked to both 'accepting' her impairment and self-identifying as a disabled person; but, having reached a point of accepting her impairment, this had enabled her to move forward.

Born with cerebral palsy, Philippa described periodically experiencing a sense of loss which she attributed to having not had the same life opportunities as her able-bodied friends. Likewise, other women with congenital impairments spoke of having experienced a sense of loss in relation to different stages of their lives such as forming relationships, getting married and having children, all of which were perceived as being the 'normal' things to do. Similarly, women who grew up with siblings of a similar age felt their 'loss' had stemmed from witnessing things that siblings (or for a small minority, friends) were doing or experiencing for example, first boyfriends or attending a school disco, yet feeling the same opportunities were denied them by virtue of their impairment.

Although born with her impairment and having used a wheelchair for mobilising from an early age, Carly spoke of living through childhood with the hope that she would one day walk but considered herself to have experienced loss when confronted with the reality that her impairment was to be a permanent fixture of her life:

> Although I was born with my condition growing up I always felt that it was something I would grow out of ... there were people at school who sometimes used a wheelchair but other days would walk and I thought that could be me though I don't know exactly why. I think I was about 12 when I realised it was a mad dream and that my wheelchair was for life ... I had a tough few months when I rallied against stuff ... it just felt like a loss ... but six years on I'm ok now it's just how things are and I manage ok.
>
> Carly (age 18, congenital impairment)

As the oldest participant Elisabeth had experienced loss at different stages of her life which had stemmed from both declines in her physical abilities and the premature death of her husband from cancer. As periodic declines in her progressive impairment occurred, Elisabeth recalled striving to adapt to her changed circumstances but that overall this had been an unconscious process and like other women did not identify with going through stages of adjustment, at the end of which she considered herself 'recovered'.

Loss: Additional Aspects

Within a study which explored the issue of loss among a group of wheelchair-users, Sapey (1996) highlighted a number of areas within people's lives other than their impairment in which loss may be experienced such as losing control of what happened after onset of impairment and being excluded from, or not fully involved in fundamental decisions for example, about home adaptations to accommodate their needs or what form of care package would be provided. Having no active involvement in decisions that were made by health and social care professionals despite having full mental capacity, was shown within Sapey's study to have been a source of frustration for many individuals and for the majority had constituted a significant area of loss of control. Of interest from my own study data (Smith 2010) was evidence of contrasting opinions relating to transition to wheelchair use for two women and whilst the transition from using a manual chair to a powered wheelchair had represented to Lisa a decline in her physical ability, it was interpreted as having enabled greater independence and thus was not experienced as a 'loss'. In contrast, Maria had experienced losing the ability to walk and becoming a full-time wheelchair-user as devastating and had endured great difficulty in coming to terms with losing the ability to drive with the subsequent loss of independence having resulted in an acute sense of loss.

A further area of loss highlighted by Sapey (2004), and one which he claimed to be seldom recognised by professionals, was the price that disabled individuals will often have to pay with regard to a general loss of privacy and an increased vulnerability in order to receive care services, and was indeed spoken of by a number of the study participants. Lisa, for example, described a review assessment of her care package in which the visiting social worker explained that budget cuts meant that services could only be offered to those with the greatest needs:

> When the social worker came to check if I still needed the care they were providing it was a horrible experience … it was like you had to portray yourself in a really negative way … say how bad things were and what terrible things might happen if that help was taken away … it was really degrading … having to fight for something that has to be there because of your physical condition and not something you would want through choice let's face it.
>
> Lisa (age 45, congenital impairment)

Similar experiences were shared by women with acquired impairments who, having lost their previously able-bodied status, were confronted with situations in which both their privacy and dignity had often been compromised. For two women, the process of applying for disability benefits which had involved both lengthy medical examinations and a requirement to provide written accounts of their dependent needs had been experienced as both upsetting and humiliating and perceived as reinforcing the stereotypes of disabled people as helpless and dependent which conversely in recent decades, society has been making steps to shift away from.

Over recent years, one of the criticisms directed at the literature concerned with loss has been the lack of consideration for whether loss, where experienced, is done so differently for women (and men) born with their impairments and those who acquire them. People who acquire an impairment (in particular where the onset is rapid), French (1994) believed would be more likely than people with congenital impairments or those who develop their impairments more slowly, to feel an acute sense of loss. Likewise, women with acquired impairments were felt more likely to undertake a process of transition whilst they experience a shift both in their own position, and in that of people around them, a view which was supported by data evidence. Having previously lived as an able-bodied person, French believed that those who acquire an impairment would be more likely to comprehend their disadvantaged status in society than individuals whose impairments were present at birth and would have had to learn how to operate as a disabled person.

Working with Disabled Clients in Counselling: Counselling Approaches

In addition to the emergence of alternative approaches to loss which claim to offer a more realistic portrayal of how disabled people adjust to or live with their impairments, criticisms directed at loss approaches led to demands for counselling approaches that both recognise the potential for oppression within the counsellor–client relationship and which utilise the social model of disability as a key foundation of their work with disabled clients (Corker 2004, Tew 2011, Machin 2013). A number of counselling approaches which have been suggested may be helpful when working with disabled clients will now be considered.

Person-centred Counselling

Within literature which has examined the topic area of counselling and disabled people, the use of *person-centred counselling* which makes no assumption about how individuals respond to disability and impairment has increasingly been proposed for disabled women (and men) who have been assessed as needing, or who have expressed a wish for counselling support. In contrast to loss approaches to counselling, advocates of person-centred counselling claim that the approach encourages people to explore and express their own thoughts and feelings without intervention or evaluation by the counsellor (Lenny 1993, Wilson 2003, Reeve 2004) whilst also being favoured for emphasising client power above authoritarian power and advocating collaborative power in the client counsellor relationship (Mearns and Thorne 1999, Nattiello 2001). A person-centred approach has also been advocated for the way in which the counsellor and client relationship is at its core (Johnson 2011) with the process also involving the art of encounter where both parties aim to operate from a position of power from within (Casemore 2006). According to Johnson, where disabled clients are involved, this may mean easing out anxieties and fears so that both parties can come into closer connection with each other and may also involve the counsellor reaching out and noticing when the client appears ashamed or presents as being unable to talk about distressing experiences. Whilst it is important for the counsellor to be informed by the client about their experience of living with disability, in addition to her/his responses to that, Johnson (2011) believes that counsellors or allied professionals who provide counselling as part of their role in working with disabled people, cannot understand people's experiences in their entirety until people let them know what those experiences are.

A person-centred approach to working with disabled clients has additionally being favoured for the specific emphasis placed on the counsellors' capacity to address their own fears, anxieties and prejudices whilst additionally being aware of working within a social and cultural context that is often oppressive of disabled people. By counsellors becoming aware of their own positioning as counsellors in addition to acknowledging that positioning in relationships with clients is an ongoing process, Olkin (1999) claims will assist the counselling process for both parties.

Evidence from the research and similarly highlighted by Paulson et al. (2007) was how the counselling approach utilised by the counsellor was often linked to an individual's rating of the counselling process's effectiveness in addressing their mental distress. Lisa described her experience of undergoing counselling in which a person-centred approach was utilised:

> When I first started those counselling sessions I couldn't get along with the person-centred approach and felt it wasn't going to work … I think I'd gone along expecting the counsellor to do the talking and to have the answers and I found the long silences quite stressful … I came to realise that the counsellor wanted to hear things from me … how things were from my perspective and it was different to what I'd experienced before.
>
> Lisa (age 45, congenital impairment)

As her counselling progressed, Lisa spoke of recognising the approach's benefit but that the limited number of sessions had resulted in the overall process not being viewed very positively and as having provided limited benefit in improving her mental well-being.

Cognitive Counselling

In calling for counselling approaches which it is claimed will make therapy services more accessible to disabled people who express a wish for, or are identified as potentially benefiting from counselling (Triskel, Jade et al. 2007), the use of a *cognitive approach* has been considered to be a useful one. Within a cognitive approach, damaging thinking patterns such as disabled people telling themselves they are hopeless, lacking intelligence and unattractive are confronted, with the counsellor giving assistance in replacing these with more positive thoughts. In particular, a cognitive approach, French (1994) believed, may benefit individuals who, through a variety of life experiences which may or not be associated with their impairment, may have developed low self-esteem and self-confidence. Additionally, advocates of cognitive counselling believe it to be an approach that may assist and encourage disabled people to act on their own behalf through expression of their feelings, needs and desires in a way that is both self-assured and confident. Having worked with a counsellor who utilised a cognitive approach, Helen recalled its impact on the counselling process overall:

> The counsellor I've been seeing for some months, did what nobody has done before ... he explained how different approaches were used, often depending on the person and what their issues are ... and he explained what cognitive counselling was ... as the sessions have continued and I'm hoping to reduce the frequency soon I've seen how the approach has worked really well for me and has improved my self-esteem and confidence and helped me to think more positively overall.
>
> Helen (age 41, congenital impairment)

Similarly, Judith believed she had benefited from the counsellor's use of a cognitive approach:

> When I eventually started counselling I hadn't really thought about how the process worked I was just glad that at last I was getting to talk to someone ... that said I knew some of the basics about cognitive counselling as we had a speaker at the stroke support group who spoke to us about counselling. I remember when I started my sessions I was quite down in myself and just felt worthless ... like I couldn't do anything anymore, couldn't work ... But the counsellor over the weeks helped me turn those negative thoughts around ... mainly by looking at things in a different way.
>
> Judith (age 61, acquired paralysis following stroke)

Through establishing changes in her thought processes, Judith described how cognitive counselling had, and continued to enable her to view things differently. When now experiencing periods of feeling down Judith spoke of being able to apply what she had learned through counselling to turn negative thoughts or feelings into more positive ones which, in turn, positively affected her overall mental well-being.

In a study that looked at the use of cognitive behavioural therapy (CBT) with a focus on specific practical problem-solving techniques, the mood of everyone in a group of individuals living with Multiple Sclerosis was found to have improved significantly (Dennison et al. 2010) with other small scale studies showing a marked decline in clinical depression among people living with MS when CBT was used (Larocco 2000, Siegert and Abernethy 2005). Current NICE guidelines for people living with Multiple Sclerosis are seen to encourage initially a self-management approach to tackling depression, stating that eating healthily, sleeping well and using positive coping strategies can all help to improve mood with exercise additionally emphasised as being an important factor in triggering endorphins, the body's natural anti-depressant (Multiple Sclerosis Society 2011). Research has also shown clinical depression to be the most common and likely psychological change to be experienced in the months following a stroke with The Stroke Association estimating that approximately half of stroke survivors will be diagnosed with depression, and likewise emphasising the likely benefits of following a healthy diet and undertaking physical exercise (The Stroke Association 2012). However, such guidelines have attracted criticism for their failure to acknowledge that people living with Multiple Sclerosis, a stroke, a spinal injury or other neurological conditions which to varying degrees may affect mobility and functional abilities, may be unable to undertake any physical exercise of note, with quality of sleep a luxury that may be craved but denied by virtue of the effects of a person's condition such as pain, spasms or fatigue (Smith 2003). Similarly, the research (Smith 2010) demonstrated how, for some women, positive approaches to coping had in recent years been increasingly hampered by anxieties over issues such as changes to welfare benefits and ad hoc reassessments of eligibility for care and support services. When confronted with such uncertainties, several women commented on how advice to 'stay positive' was felt to be patronising and thus creating feelings of frustration and upset and subsequently potentially exacerbating mental distress (Smith 2010).

The use of *cognitive approaches* have been contrasted with the use of *behavioural approaches* which Lenny (1993) strongly rejected for use with disabled clients. Based on their assumptions that any problems that an individual encounters arise from within themselves as opposed to within society, Lenny claimed such approaches equate to those of a medical model approach in which the individual's 'disability' was 'the problem'. The use of a behavioural approach by Elisabeth's counsellor had been experienced as unhelpful through having reinforced her feelings of self-blame for the mental and psychological distress she was experiencing and which, through counselling Elisabeth had wished to reverse. Conversely, a cognitive approach utilised by a different counsellor had proved a more positive experience in which she had been enabled to explore her negative thoughts and with assistance given in replacing them with more positive ones:

> I was at a low ebb when I started counselling but assumed the counsellor knew best, he explained about the different approaches but as I was so down at the time the theory side of stuff I didn't think about much … but over time the behavioural approach seemed to reinforce my thoughts of being to blame for anything that had gone wrong … like it was all my fault … eventually I sought private counselling which was expensive and took a long time to find someone who I thought was suitable as I couldn't find a disabled counsellor anywhere but the cognitive approach they used even after a few weeks things seemed better and improved my mental well-being quite a bit.
>
> Elisabeth (age 62, congenital impairment)

Disability Counselling Approaches

In acknowledging the importance of cultural differences between the counsellor and the client and the effect that this has on counselling practice, within *trans-cultural counselling* (TCC), counsellors work across cultural boundaries, accepting that there is a world view other than their own. Likewise, in recognising both the potentially oppressive aspects of counselling and any issues of prejudice and discrimination in the client's life, these are also perceived to be appropriate areas to consider when working with disabled clients (McLeod 1998). In particular, trans-cultural counselling is felt to address any cultural and racial prejudices of the counsellor and how they affect the counsellor–client relationship, thus, many of the issues covered by TCC such as the reality of prejudice and discrimination in the life of the client are also claimed to be appropriate issues to consider when working with disabled clients (D'Ardenne 1999, 2013). However, whilst considered to be an approach that may be useful when working with disabled clients, Reeve does not consider TCC in its present form to offer a complete solution for working with disabled clients given that disabled people are not a homogenous group and like able-bodied people are likely to be living alone, within families or within communities of non-disabled people. Therefore, in seeking to provide counselling approaches which both recognise the potentially oppressive nature of counselling and seek to redress the power imbalance between the counsellor and disabled client, Reeve (2006) has proposed two possible solutions.

Firstly, the creation of a *disability counselling* approach which both recognises oppression within the counselling room and which incorporates the social model of disability as its cornerstone is advocated. Like TCC, Reeve (2006) claims that disability counselling would be profoundly social and political as well as personal and individual, and additionally would challenge disablist attitudes and prejudices in the same way that trans-cultural counselling challenges institutional racism within the counsellor. Disability Counselling, likewise, would be aware of the connection between social context alongside an expectation that the counsellor would look at disability from a social model perspective whilst also assisting disabled clients to move away from blaming themselves for being socially excluded. Whilst acknowledging that not all disabled people consider themselves to be 'disabled' or prefer the use of alternative terminology for example, less able, differently abled or as having impaired mobility, counselling from a social model perspective Reeve believes would be preferable to ignoring the reality of oppression both within and outside of the counselling room environment. Furthermore, professional training for a disability counselling approach would place a strong emphasis on self-awareness work on the part of the counsellor in order to address attitudes, beliefs and stereotypes about disabled people and disability which may have been instilled within them since pre adulthood and never been questioned (Reeve 2006).

A second proposed approach draws attention to counselling approaches which, since the turn of the century, have adopted a social and political rather than a psychological stance. Aspiring to achieve comprehensive, anti-oppressive practice that offers empowering counselling for all individuals irrespective of race, gender, class or impairment, advocates claim that these counselling approaches potentially have much to offer to people with physical (and visual and sensory) impairments as well as other oppressed and disadvantaged groups within society (Swain, Griffiths and Heyman 2003). Within the newly emerging approaches significant emphasis is placed on counsellors receiving training in areas which recognise the totality of human experiences: the political, social and historical contexts in addition to the psychological aspects and whilst social approaches to counselling are evolving, the importance of disability as a socially created oppression rather than an individual tragedy to be represented and included from the outset is also emphasised. In so doing, such approaches are considered more likely to meet the needs of disabled people rather than leaving it to health and social care professionals who work with disabled clients to make assumptions about their needs, on their behalf (Reeve 2006).

However, in advocating alternative counselling approaches for disabled people, their potential to be divisive is acknowledged with Reeve (2006) therefore questioning whether another way of differentiating between disabled people and able-bodied people is either wanted or needed. Research by Oliver (1995) which considered whether a specific model of counselling was needed to help disabled people cope with the emotional effects of their impairment found there to be a majority belief among a group of counsellors (able-bodied and disabled) who had worked with disabled people for a minimum of three years, that disabled people did not need to be counselled in ways that were significantly different from any other group. Like other groups in society, disabled people, like their able-bodied counterparts are multifaceted through ethnicity, gender, class and sexuality and are not a homogenous group and the appropriateness of providing counselling which arguably emphasises the disabled dimension of a person is therefore questionable. Further, by proposing specific counselling approaches for disabled people, this adds to the continuing debate concerning whether those who require or seek counselling are best served by a monolithic approach which addresses specifically the concerns of disabled people, or by emerging social approaches to counselling which view clients as holistic human beings with their physical impairment but one element of their whole being. On balance, current counselling literature appears to recognise the need for disability as social oppression to be incorporated into the counselling theories that inform counselling practice. Without this, oppression in the counselling room will arguably be sustained and disabled people will be prevented from gaining worthwhile benefit from their contacts with counsellors (Reeve 2000), a view that was echoed firmly within the study's findings and which will be explored within Chapter 4.

Conclusions

This chapter began by highlighting the expansion of counselling services UK-wide through the latter decades of the twentieth century and beyond, and considered examples of specific counselling approaches which over recent decades have been used when working specifically with women. Also discussed was how some aspects of the women's counselling experiences had been positive, with the approaches used by the counsellors described as having been beneficial for some women. However, as a client group several women had felt themselves to be not well-served by counsellors who were felt to have little understanding of the lived experience of impairment or disability which in turn had impacted on women's rating of the effectiveness of counselling in treating their mental distress. Furthermore, the lack of suitable counselling approaches available to counsellors working with disabled clients and a lack of attention devoted to issues around equal opportunities within counselling training had additionally reinforced a belief in the need both for disability equality training to become a mandatory part of all training courses and likewise for increased opportunities for people with physical impairments to be able to train as counsellors.

Increasingly over the past decade, counselling responses to disability based on loss theories have been criticised for their disempowering nature and their failure to recognise the potential for oppression within the counsellor–client relationship. Whilst there had been among the sample group a shared belief that at some stage of living with their impairment they would experience loss, the ways in which loss was understood and how it was experienced had varied widely with the chapter having further illustrated how experiences of loss were attributed to factors other than impairment. Further, the chapter has shown how across the group the stages theory approach to adjusting to impairment was neither agreed nor identified with, instead women were seen to identify with more recent approaches to loss which have been proposed as offering a more realistic explanation of how disabled people live with and/or adjust to their individual impairments. In providing counselling which in future is likely to be of value to disabled people, the chapter has highlighted the argument for counselling approaches which utilise the social model of disability as one of its foundations and by moving away from the viewpoint of disability as a personal tragedy and the associated assumption that it has a negative impact on the life of the disabled person, it has been suggested will benefit all disabled clients. However, whilst a disability counselling approach has been suggested, its potential to be divisive has been openly acknowledged whilst whether a further way of differentiating between able-bodied people and disabled people is either wanted or needed has been widely questioned. The usefulness of an approach in which the main focus is the 'disabled' dimension of an individual has likewise been questioned and links arguably to the ongoing debate as to whether disabled people need to work with counsellors who themselves are disabled (or have lived-experience of impairment) or, if an able-bodied counsellor is equally well-suited to provide the counselling support that an individual requires and is a topic that will be discussed within Chapter 4.

In learning from the mixed experiences of receiving counselling which have been reported by disabled clients in recent years (Smith 2003, Morris 2004, Jack 2009), Johnson (2011) suggests there to be several ways of improving counselling practice for the disabled clients of tomorrow. Firstly, for counsellors to be aware of the attitudes and values of the culture in which we live and the impact that may have on individual work with clients is considered to be vital. Furthermore, the respect that counsellors show to disabled clients should involve being transparent about personal positioning in the cultures and society in which we live and work with a need to tease out differences on an ongoing basis where barriers occur. Calling for a greater degree of reflexivity and transparency consistent with the ethos of a favoured person centred approach, in addition Johnson (2011) called for the burden of responsibility to speak out against disablism to not be left to disabled people alone, believing some challenges to structural power to only be effective when counsellors operate as a collective and that respect for clients involves challenging any form of disablism that is encountered, whether able-bodied or disabled. Through counsellors entering into encounter with people who appear to be 'different' Johnson believes will enable counsellors to be changed through that experience and in so doing gain a greater understanding of real diversity.

Chapter 4
Gender, Disability and Mental Health

Introduction

Within this chapter the issue of gender and its considered importance within the overall counselling experience for disabled women will be discussed. Within Chapter 2, attention was drawn to the growth in the late twentieth century of the women's self-help movement that worked with the belief that support was most effectively provided by women who had shared similar experiences and in ways that appreciated and valued women's strengths and characteristics. Within the study, highlighted by the data was the preference expressed by the large majority of women to work with a female counsellor and the perceived advantages and disadvantages of counsellors being the same gender as their clients will be examined. Secondly, the chapter will discuss the recently emerged and ongoing debate both within disability studies and counselling literature as to whether or not disabled people (women or men) who require or seek counselling should be counselled by disabled counsellors (or disabled allied professionals who provide counselling as part of their work role).

Findings from the research additionally demonstrated the view that individuals with either previous lived experience of impairment (such as a temporary impairment) or who have a good awareness and understanding of issues around disability and impairment by virtue of for example, having cared for or supported significantly a disabled person may be suitable candidates to work with disabled clients. Thus, the considered likely advantages or otherwise of disabled clients working with counsellors or other mental health professionals with lived-experience of impairment who may provide counselling as part of their work role with disabled clients will be discussed in addition to considering other factors or attributes which women felt were important for a counsellor to be able to offer or exhibit. Evidenced by the study were the difficulties that women had encountered in locating a disabled counsellor and the availability of disabled counsellors UK-wide will be discussed. Finally, the chapter will consider women's accounts of their experiences of mental distress and the factors which, at a personal level, were considered to have been significant within those experiences.

Women and Counselling: The Effect of Gender

Within Chapter 3 the expansion of counselling approaches which, in the later decades of the twentieth century were advocated as considering the specific needs and circumstances of women and which were felt to best be provided by counsellors of the same gender, were discussed. Within a small study which examined the personal experiences of using mental health services for eight disabled women, a key finding was the preferred wish of all women to have had the opportunity to work in counselling with a female counsellor or other mental health professional who provides counselling as part of their work role (Smith 2003). In seeking to explore further any reasons or rationale for such preferences, within the recent study (Smith 2010) women were asked to share any personal preferences held for working with a counsellor or allied professional of a specific gender. Within the sample group, all women had received counselling on at least one occasion with five women having worked with counsellors on more than four occasions. Whilst five women had worked both with female and male counsellors, six had worked only with female counsellors and one woman who received counselling twice, had worked on both occasions with a hospital-based male psychologist. However, across the group just two women expressed a preference to work in counselling with a male counsellor, with 10 having cited a preference to work with a female counsellor or allied professional, where counselling was deemed to be necessary or being sought through personal choice, the majority preferences shown to primarily have been explained by a perception of feeling more at ease talking to a counsellor or allied professional of the same gender.

Within the sample group, women who had worked with female counsellors recalled experiencing initial anxieties at the start of their counselling but that counsellors had helped at an early stage of the process to put them at ease which had then remained and had assisted the counselling process overall. With similar thoughts and views expressed by other women, Philippa described her sense of relief when allocated to a female counsellor:

> I've had counselling a few times now during the times I've been really depressed … both with a counsellor and a psychiatric nurse and each time you get referred you don't know whether it will be a man or a woman and seems you don't get to choose. So when I get the call or letter and realise it's a woman it does settle the anxiety while I'm waiting to find out. … but the counselling itself, I would always choose a female just because stuff you talk about often is really personal and can be hard to talk about so you have to feel as relaxed as you can be and comfortable … I can't put an exact finger on it just that I feel I can relate better to a woman and that I could open up in a way I don't feel I could with a male counsellor … that said I haven't experienced working with a male counsellor so I can't really make a comparison.
>
> Philippa (age 36, congenital impairment)

Likewise, data provided evidence of a shared belief amongst six women that if the issues being addressed within counselling were associated with gender and/or gender roles, that a female counsellor would have a better understanding of, and/or insight into what the woman was experiencing as was highlighted by Elisabeth:

> The first time I went for counselling I was hoping it would be a woman, I knew it wouldn't be anyone who [was] disabled as I'd already hit a brick wall with that already … I felt I would work better with a female not just because I thought I'd feel more at ease though and even that I knew there'd be no guarantee but it was mainly because at that time my distress was linked to issues around being a woman … it's hard to explain exactly but I just felt personally that a male counsellor would be unlikely to have the insight that a woman would.
>
> Elisabeth (age 62, congenital impairment)

Upon completion of her counselling sessions, Elisabeth recalled how there remained issues she needed to continue to work on, building on what she had learned through the counselling process but mentally considered herself to be much improved and which to a significant extent was attributed to having worked with a female counsellor with whom she had been able to establish with relative ease a good working relationship. Elisabeth further commented on how a later experience of working with a male counsellor had proved to be more positive than she had anticipated but believed this to have been a consequence of the issues being addressed within counselling on that occasion having not been linked directly to her gender.

In contrast, the preference of two women to work in counselling with a male professional was based on the reality in their everyday lives of getting on better with males than females. Both recalled in their counselling sessions having forged with relative ease a good working relationship with their male counsellor which had assisted in enabling them to talk openly about their mental distress. Frankie described her experience:

> Overall my preference would always be to work with a male counsellor as generally I tend to get on better with men than women I'm not sure why … when I went to my first counselling appointment it was a woman but I wasn't unduly bothered and was happy to give things a go but as time progressed I just felt it wasn't working and we clashed on a number of levels … as I sensed it wasn't working it affected my motivation to commit to the sessions so I asked to switch to another counsellor which I didn't think they'd agree to but they did and the chap I was allocated to, well the counselling was a lot better, the whole experience was.
>
> Frankie (age 27, congenital impairment)

Whilst being aware of the requirement for all counsellors to be non-judgmental in undertaking their work with all clients, Helen had encountered female counsellors whom she considered to have been judgmental of how she perceived different areas of her life:

> I felt that when I worked with female counsellors they could be judgmental of some of my thought processes … I know my mind was quite fixed about certain

> things and I found it hard to consider alternative points of view especially when I was quite unwell but it did affect the counselling sessions and for me personally … I've just found that male counsellors are more willing to listen and had more patience with me because listening can be difficult with my speech problems.
>
> Helen (age 41, congenital impairment)

Helen's preference to work with male counsellors was also partly attributed to the poor relationships which she had with her sisters growing up which contrasted with a strong relationship with an elder brother who had provided ongoing emotional support:

> Even as a young girl I remember not getting on with my sisters, feeling they resented me because of the extra help and attention I needed and I think my quite poor and strained relationships with my sisters have been a part of my preference to work with male health or social care professionals generally … it's always been my brother I've gone to when I've been upset and he was there for me when I was diagnosed with breast cancer.
>
> Helen (age 41, congenital impairment)

Whilst specific gender preferences were expressed group-wide, women acknowledged that the opportunity to work with a counsellor or professional of gender choice provided no automatic guarantee of establishing a good working relationship. Attributes such as a counsellor's personality or character traits were thus considered to be potentially significant in contributing to a counselling process that was perceived to have addressed effectively a woman's mental or psychological distress and in which the outcome was viewed positively.

Having previously worked with female counsellors, four women commented on how prior to entering into counselling their personal preferences would have been to work with a female counsellor primarily for the reasons cited above, and that if allocated to a male professional, to varying degrees women would have considered that the counselling process was unlikely to have positive or beneficial outcomes. In addition, study data provided evidence of a shared perception that neither a male counsellor's listening skills nor their ability to empathise with the mental distress a woman was experiencing could match those of their female counterparts, and particularly so if the nature or origin of the woman's distress was linked to their gender.

Lisa described her underlying feelings during the initial counselling sessions with a male counsellor:

> I've been with my husband for 15 years and have lost count of the times I've said to him … you don't listen, you don't understand and I just assumed I'd feel the same way about a male counsellor … but actually as time went on I came to realise that you can't assume every man is incapable of listening or unwilling to understand. I gradually relaxed and felt able to talk to him though and overall

> the experience was worthwhile and whilst I still think my preference if I needed counselling again would be for a female counsellor the prospect of working with a male one would no longer worry me unduly.
>
> Lisa (age 45, congenital impairment)

Having received counselling from numerous mental health professionals over a period of two decades linked to both her clinical depression and eating distress, Claire similarly recalled her reality of working with a male counsellor for over a year to have differed widely from her expectations and considered the process to have been the most positive of several counselling experiences:

> About 10 years ago I went through a bad episode with my eating distress and was referred to a therapist whose specialism was working with people with eating disorders ... I went along assuming it would be a woman as I guess you associate women more with eating disorders so was a bit taken aback when a chap introduced himself. For a while I had quite low expectations as I couldn't see how a man could understand this sort of stuff and often I came close to cancelling appointments ... But over time I realised that although he hadn't experienced eating distress personally his understanding of issues around it was really good plus he was an excellent listener and totally non-judgmental. ... it took a long time to get to where I wanted to be but the outcomes eventually were definitely positive and I went back to work in much better shape physically and mentally.
>
> Claire (age 39, acquired spinal illness)

Whilst the study highlighted a preference for the majority of the women to work with female counsellors, the reality had been that unless counselling was privately funded a choice was very unlikely to be offered or available. The issue of disabled clients being offered a choice of gender will be discussed further within Chapter 5.

Disabled Counsellors for Disabled People?

Within counselling literature of recent years the emergence and growth of a debate among counsellors, disabled people and disabled academics as to whether or not disabled people should only be counselled by disabled counsellors has been evident (Reeve 2004, Bryant-Jeffries 2004). In a study which examined counsellors' perspectives of counselling disabled people (Oliver 1995), whilst some counsellors suggested that a disabled counsellor may be too subjective or too close having had lived experience of disability and/or impairment, others felt that a non-disabled counsellor may be too objective or distant having had no personal experience of living as a disabled person. Whilst it was suggested that an able-bodied counsellor could be accused of being unable to comprehend what it is like to live as a disabled person, and therefore would have no understanding of the needs of this client group, some counsellors felt that no two impairments or experience of those impairments would ever be identical and that by the very nature of the profession, a good counsellor should be able to empathise with another person whatever the issues raised or differences in life experiences (Oliver 1995).

Within a previous study which examined the experiences of mental distress and of accessing mental health services for eight disabled women (Smith 2003), the group-wide preferences to work with a disabled counsellor were based on a belief that a disabled counsellor would have a greater understanding and awareness of disability issues, with one woman particularly keen to work with a counsellor who was *both* female and disabled, believing that this would enable a wholly positive counselling experience. Counsellors and allied professionals from whom the women had received counselling i.e. community psychiatric nurses, were perceived overall to have been unfamiliar with physical impairment and as having little or no previous contact with disabled clients (Smith 2003) with similar views expressed by participants within Morris's (2004) study which examined mental health provision for people with physical impairments.

Just as analysed data suggested there to be no right or wrong answer as to whether a same gender counsellor or mental health professional was likely to be the person best suited to work with a disabled woman (or man), this was equally apparent in relation to whether a disabled counsellor (or one with lived experience of impairment) was the most appropriate individual to work with disabled individuals who experience mental distress. Evidence from both the interview and focus group data highlighted diverse views concerning the perceived advantages and disadvantages of working with a counsellor or allied professional with personal experience of impairment (or a good knowledge, understanding and awareness by virtue of for example, being a long-term carer of a disabled family member) as opposed to an able-bodied counsellor with minimal experience or understanding of impairment.

With all 12 women having received professional counselling on one or more occasions, seven would have welcomed the opportunity to work with a disabled counsellor, with a majority view expressed that a disabled counsellor (or one with lived experience of impairment) would in particular be beneficial if the issues to be addressed within counselling were related to their impairment. Having acquired a spinal injury at the age of 13, Jackie outlined the benefits she had derived from talking with patients who were experiencing similar psychological difficulties to her own in adjusting to their altered mobility and changed life circumstances and believing overall that a counsellor (preferably with an acquired impairment), would be best suited to provide counselling to individuals with acquired impairments who either expressed a wish for, or were identified as needing professional counselling. Whilst acknowledging the essentiality of counsellors undergoing professional training in order to be able to offer appropriate and professional support, Jackie believed that some level of personal experience (either direct or indirect) was required in order to have a full understanding and appreciation of living as a disabled person. However, several women emphasised the need for disabled counsellors to acknowledge that although there may be similarities in the ways in which women (and men) live with their impairments, ultimately, and as referred to above each individual's experience will be unique to them. Similarly, within a study that examined experiences of the counselling process from the perspective of a number of disabled clients (Jack 2009), the most positive counselling experiences were reported in instances where the counsellor had personal experience of living as a disabled person or, had a good understanding of and insight into impairment and disability by virtue of currently being, or having previously been, a primary carer for a disabled person.

For Morris, an expressed wish for a disabled counsellor may be because of the shared experience of impairment and disability, in contrast to an expressed preference by some disabled people for a non-disabled counsellor which may have resulted result from an internalised oppression which has instilled a personal belief that a disabled counsellor will not be as good as an able-bodied counsellor (Morris 2004). However, women within the study's focus group were not seen to support this view and whilst Reeve (2004) did not consider it to be necessary for disabled people to be counselled by disabled counsellors, a greater availability of disabled counsellors within the counselling professions she believed would improve client choice for individuals who expressed a preference to work with a disabled counsellor. Currently within the UK, for most disabled people seeking a disabled counsellor, the current scarcity means that choice is rarely an option; whilst Skylark (London-based), Mosaic (Leicester-based) and Spokz people (Midlands-based) are rare examples of organisations which provide counselling to, and are managed and staffed by disabled people, such services are often geographically localised and available only to disabled people living within those areas and services may not be free of charge.

Four women recalled how the issues which they had addressed within their counselling sessions had primarily been concerned with relationship breakdowns or difficulties or financial or work concerns and these women therefore considered that an able-bodied counsellor may be equally well-suited to provide appropriate counselling support. A recent experience of psychological distress had, for Jackie resulted from difficulty in coming to terms with finishing paid work, but in not perceiving her distress to be linked *directly* to her impairment had not felt a need to work with a disabled counsellor (and believed that her chances of being offered the opportunity) were minimal. A positive experience of working with an able-bodied counsellor who systematically worked through with Jackie the circumstances surrounding her emotional distress, had enabled her to recognise that whilst finishing paid employment represented a change in her physical health, it simultaneously provided new opportunities to pursue other areas of work interests but with a flexibility that matched her physical limitations.

However, caution of this view was expressed by some women, in particular Alison who stressed the need for a consideration of whether the difficulties that had led to a need for counselling either had their origins in, or were indirectly linked to the woman's impairment, and that lived experience of impairment may therefore remain advantageous:

> My first counselling experience was after the break-up of my marriage and I was struggling to cope. The counsellor was an able-bodied woman and at the time I didn't really think it mattered that she was able-bodied … but as time went on because she had no experience of disability I came to realise that she couldn't see how or the ways in which my disability had a knock-on effect on my relationship with my husband and eventually led to us breaking up.
>
> Alison (age 38, congenital impairment)

Similarly, whilst lived experience of physical impairment was not considered to be a pre-requisite of being able to provide effective counselling to disabled women (or men) either in need of or seeking counselling, both a good understanding of disability and impairment and insight into how an individual's impairment may potentially impact on different areas of their life were considered to be of great importance. Whilst Alison's first counselling experience was considered to have been ineffective in treating her mental distress, a second more positive experience was attributed to the able-bodied, female counsellor having a similar socio-economic background to her own and having both grown up within farming communities Alison perceived the counsellor to have both a good understanding of, and an empathy with the difficulties she was experiencing. Prior to entering into counselling, Alison believed that if a choice between working with an able-bodied or disabled counsellor had been offered, her preference would have been the latter and that her initial expectations of working for a second time with an able-bodied counsellor had been low. However, the counsellors similar socio-economic background had proved for Alison to be invaluable and alerted her to a realisation that attributes or factors other than a physical impairment per se may be as, or more important in providing optimum opportunity for a positive counselling relationship in which the set agreed goals between counsellor and client were achieved:

> After a bad experience of working with an able-bodied counsellor I was convinced second time around it would have to be someone who was disabled themselves … but working with this counsellor we just seemed to click and coming from a farming community herself she had great empathy which I think contributed a lot to a positive experience … the goals we set between us were reached and the distress I'd been going through was resolved … not entirely but enough for me to build on and move forward.
>
> Alison (age 38, congenital impairment)

Disabled Counsellors: Does a Choice Exist?

Whilst the study highlighted the preference of seven of the 12 women to work with a counsellor with lived-experience of impairment (or with someone who by virtue of their circumstances had a good understanding and awareness of issues around disability and impairment), the stark reality had been that a choice between working with a disabled counsellor and an able-bodied one seldom existed. Whilst the expansion of counselling over recent decades has resulted in a steady increase in the number of counsellors in training, the number of disabled (or trainee disabled counsellors) has by comparison remained consistently low (Reeve 2004) with none of the women having been offered the opportunity to work with a counsellor with lived experience of impairment. According to Corker, people with physical impairments wish to become counsellors for the same reasons as able-bodied people, for example, wishing to provide support to people experiencing difficulties in their lives and believing they have the necessary skills and qualities to do so. Alternatively, the desire to become a counsellor may be associated with past personal experience of receiving counselling, or, having listened to others recollecting their negative counselling experiences, in having a wish to improve counselling experiences for others in future years (Corker 2004). Historically, the high cost of counselling training courses combined with inaccessible teaching venues in particular prior to the Disability Discrimination Act, and/or course materials may, according to Reeve (2000) have potentially contributed to the exclusion of disabled people who wished and had the potential to train as professional counsellors. Likewise, a growing requirement over recent years for counselling courses to become accredited and recognised academically has led to increasing numbers of courses being offered within university settings with entry requirements stipulating a first degree and thus potentially excluding disabled people who may have been unable to access Higher Education.

Within the study two women spoke of their previous desires to train as a professional counsellor, each believing that their personal dual experiences of mental distress and physical impairment would have enabled them to empathise with clients whilst also providing them with a positive and worthwhile counselling experience. In similar terms, Alison and Helen explained how their access to professional training courses in the early 1990s had been hindered by a lack of academic qualifications, having been educated within special schools which had offered few opportunities to study for recognised academic qualifications. In addition, Alison's lived experiences of physical impairment and mental distress combined with her personal experiences of undergoing counselling were felt to have seemingly been disregarded throughout the application process:

> When I looked into training to become a counsellor I hit a brick wall at every turn as they all wanted qualifications in maths, english etc. with good grades. I'd always gone to special school where there hadn't been the opportunity to study for O levels because you weren't expected to go on and achieve anything … I did go on to college and got some qualifications but these weren't really taken account of. At a couple of places I got an initial interview which themselves were difficult as I wasn't really used to formal interviews so I probably didn't come across well but I did try to focus on what I could offer given my personal experiences of living with a disability and being mentally unwell as well as having had counselling a number of times but what they really wanted was a

> piece of paper that said you could read and add up numbers and it seemed like experience counted for nothing.
>
> Alison (age 38, congenital impairment)

The difficulties which Helen (and other women) had encountered in their extensive efforts to find a counsellor with lived experience of physical impairment had resulted in them sharing Reeve's view (2004) in calling for a greater availability UK-wide of disabled counsellors of both sexes:

> When my time-limited counselling on the NHS came to an end twice I felt we'd hardly scratched the surface in talking through the psychological problems I was having and felt that both therapists couldn't get to grips with stuff around my disability so tried to look for someone who specialised in working with disabled people just to see if that made a difference ... I looked within about a 30-mile radius of my home town and found counsellors in every specialism but physical disability which in itself raised all sorts of questions for me ... eventually I got a recommendation but it turned out he worked from an old converted house that had five steps to the front door and with no wheelchair accessible entrance ... you couldn't have made it up but then maybe the therapists lack of access awareness spoke volumes ... it was very disappointing.
>
> Helen (age 41, congenital impairment)

Having also searched unsuccessfully, Elisabeth recalled the response with which she was met when looking for a disabled counsellor:

> The first time I went for counselling my GP referred me ... I remember phoning up some weeks later to ask if I could be allocated to someone who was themselves disabled as I thought that would be better for me. Well the line went quiet for ages and then she said that they didn't have any counsellors with any form of disability and that she had never heard of a disabled person being able to work as a counsellor ... she even said that counsellors were there for people like disabled people which really upset me. I could hardly believe it ... Of course back 20 years ago there weren't the options to search for things or people that we have today ... it was basically the yellow pages and a phone but even with so many more options now to look for say a disabled counsellor I sadly don't think the outcome would be much different.
>
> Elisabeth (age 62, congenital impairment)

Whilst group-wide there was a consensus that it may not be necessary for all disabled people either seeking or needing counselling to work with a disabled counsellor, and likewise that some disabled people may not wish to, women concurred that an increased availability of disabled counsellors across the UK would serve to improve client choice for those whose preference was to work with a disabled counsellor or one with lived experience of impairment. Both women described how increased opportunities in recent years to undertake foundation counselling courses through a variety of routes had enabled them to successfully complete An Introduction to Counselling Training Course with the intention of proceeding in the not too distant future to the next level.

Drawing attention to a current underrepresentation of disabled therapists within the counselling profession, Jack (2009) further emphasised the importance of examining whether recruitment procedures are currently welcoming of this trainee group and highlighting the need for a greater availability of information about possible sources of funding, for example the Disabled Students Allowance, alongside a willingness of training providers to offer reasonable adjustments under the Equality Act (2010). By promoting more widely information relating to counselling training within UK disability publications such as *Disability Now* and on widely-used disability websites, women believed could be viable ways of encouraging more disabled people to consider the possibilities of becoming qualified counsellors. In addition, it was felt that the presence of counselling training professionals and helpful information relating to studying for a couselling qualification would be beneficial at UK shows, for example, Naidex UK or the Mobility Roadshow, where disabled people are the key audience, as it would provide an opportunity to talk in person with the relevant people. In striving to make progress, Jack (2009) further highlighted the need for measures to be taken to maximise an individual's potential and for disabled trainees to be retained by ensuring any reasonable adjustments are made to accommodate any individual needs with support given by course providers both in finding and undertaking placements in line with the person's chosen area of interest.

In scenarios where a disabled person is working as a counsellor, attention was drawn by Webbe (2010) to dilemmas that may require some personal consideration. Writing of her experiences as a counsellor whose physical impairment was clearly visible to others, Webbe spoke of 'the elephant in the room' and questioned whether when advertising her services or speaking with potential clients, if her wheelchair-user status should be made known. However, simultaneously she questioned why it should even be a factor to consider given the unlikelihood of there being an expectation within any form of self-advertisements or publicity material for one's skin colour, sexuality or religion to be included. Describing the look of surprise which she perceived to often register in a client's eyes at their initial introductions when confronted with a wheelchair-user counsellor, Webbe recalled a client who after three counselling sessions ceased contact due to the client having considered their own difficulties to be trivial compared to those of her own, by which Webbe presumed to mean her physical impairment. Whilst having worked effectively for a number of years with many able-bodied clients, Webbe (2010) drew attention to the dichotomy that whilst it was considered the norm for disabled people to work with able-bodied counsellors, with no questions asked about whether disabled individuals were comfortable with doing so, the issue of able-bodied people, and in particular any thoughts, feelings or prejudices they may have around working with a disabled counsellor are rarely considered. However, a feeling of 'being better off than the counsellor' may not be a perception solely of able-bodied clients, with one participant within Jack's study (2009) having discontinued their peer counselling with a disabled counsellor due to them feeling it to be 'not right' to talk about their own problems in counselling with an individual who they perceived to have difficulties greater than their own to contend with, referring to the counsellors mobility being significantly more impaired than their own.

For four women who had accessed privately-funded counselling (though for two only in the short term), all spoke of having felt both more empowered and in control of the therapeutic process overall, feelings which to varying extents were felt to have been lost in other areas of their lives and therefore was viewed to be important. However, whilst counselling literature suggests private counselling to be generally more diverse in its provision and therefore enabling wider choices, the high costs that are typically involved mean that for large numbers of disabled women (and men) seeking counselling, it is an option unlikely to be open to them due to the link between poverty and disability. Thus, the need for counsellors and therapists to consider both the specific circumstances of a disabled client, and the requirements of disability discrimination legislation to make reasonable adjustments in relation to disabled people was highlighted by Jack (2009). Furthermore, privately-funded counselling sessions will often take place either within a private space of the counsellor's home or within rooms of converted older houses which are probably more likely to present access issues for anyone with a significant mobility impairment (Lago and Smith 2004). Therefore, disabled people may often have little choice except to approach familiar sources of help that are commonly provided through the NHS and which are often associated with limitations both on the approaches offered and the timescales over which they are offered as well as the settings in which they may take place (Corker 2004).

In addition there is a dearth of counsellors working with disabled people. Several women attributed this to a consequence of the minimal time devoted to the topic areas of disability and impairment within the syllabuses of counselling training courses, resulting in trainee counsellors being unable to gain an insight into, or knowledge of, the subject areas and in turn, possibly wishing to specialise in working with disabled people. Across both data sets the need for more teaching around disability and impairment to be included within the syllabus of professional training courses for counsellors and other mental health professionals who may as part of their work role provide counselling support to disabled women (and men) was clearly highlighted. A belief that an increased focus on disability and impairment would enable able-bodied counsellors to develop a greater knowledge and awareness of issues around these topic areas was evidenced clearly by the data and will be discussed within Chapter 5.

Shared Understandings not Segregated Services

Whilst seven women expressed a preference to work with a disabled counsellor (or one with lived experience or a good knowledge and understanding of impairment/disability), group-wide women were not in favour of disabled people solely being counselled by disabled counsellors or those with lived experience of impairment. In so doing, women felt this could lead potentially to a situation in which counselling services became segregated and, according to Reeve (2004) could have an emotional impact in serving to remind disabled clients that they are 'different' and thus leaving them feeling socially excluded. Further, attention was drawn by Thomas (1999) to how the psycho-emotional dimension of disability can be compounded further by counsellors who fail to treat their clients with forethought and respect, for example, by thinking to move a chair or room furniture that may present an obstacle for someone with mobility difficulties, the failure of counsellors and agencies to consider the access requirements of potential disabled clients further believed to be in part, a consequence of the low number of disabled counsellors within counselling practice. Reeve also suggests there to be a myth that disabled people are counselled 'somewhere else' by experts who have specialist counselling skills for working with this client group but believes that as anyone can become disabled at any time through accident or illness, such a myth defends a counsellor from having to look at their own fears and vulnerabilities around illness, disability or death (Reeve 2004). Further, to implement a regime in which disabled women (and men) in need of or seeking counselling had access solely to disabled counsellors, women firmly believed would represent a backward step at a point in time when within society, both awareness of, and attitudes towards disability and physical impairment were felt to be improving, and people with physical (and sensory and visual) impairments were considered to be steadily becoming more integrated within a twenty-first-century world overall.

Attention was further drawn within the study to the importance of all counsellors being trained to work with disability issues as and when the need arose. Like able-bodied people, disabled people may wish within counselling to look at childhood traumas, relationship difficulties or issues associated with impairment or disability and ultimately are seeking counselling which meets their perceived needs. Almost half of the participants described how their impairment could sometimes be accompanied by chronic or intermittent episodes of illness or pain which could lead to episodes of emotional distress. However, the need for counsellors and allied mental health and social care professionals to recognise that this was not always the case and that disabled women (and men) can be emotionally stressed in ways that were not linked to their impairment was firmly emphasised. In addition, attention was drawn to the fact that as individuals they were not just women living with physical impairments but were also parents, daughters, spouses, friends or siblings who could be subject to the same range of emotions as able-bodied women. Therefore, women felt that whilst their impairments, and any specific mental health needs relating to that needed to be recognised, they wished to have equal access to any counselling services provision for able-bodied women should those services be required.

Counselling and Communication Impairments

Within the context of their experiences of mental distress, women were asked to share any thoughts around factors aside from gender and impairment which were considered to be potentially significant within viewing the counselling experience in a positive light and with analysed data highlighting a number of issues. Firstly, the importance to all women of effective communication was clearly evident with the need for counsellors (and other professionals providing counselling as part of their work role) to both listen and pay attention to the woman's spoken words and views widely emphasised as being important in providing the optimum opportunity for a good working relationship between counsellor and client to be forged. In addition, several women spoke of how, within counselling, they wished to be treated as an individual, with a feeling of being listened to having for Lisa helped the counselling process overall:

> When I had counselling some years ago I thought at first the awkwardness was just part of getting to know them but over time we just didn't seem to click and I felt I wasn't being listened to but second time around it just felt different … as if I felt I could communicate better and things the counsellor said it just made me feel that she was really listening to the things I was saying … they didn't cut across my sentences and just gave me the time I needed to find best I could the right words.
>
> Lisa (age 45, congenital impairment)

In particular, the art of listening when working with people with communication or language impairments is for counsellors particularly important with developments in communication technology over recent years, for example, speech recognition software or communication boards having had a significant impact on the lives of some disabled people (Dalton 1994, French and Swain 2004). Whilst the psychological effects of such advances have yet in the early twenty-first century to be fully investigated and recognised, for the field of psychotherapy in which communication is the primary tool, technology has been claimed to be of particular interest for the new possibilities that it has, and continues to open up in working with individuals with speech impairments or those who rely on non-verbal communication (Sheldon 2001, Wilson 2003, Anthony and Goss 2003). Within the study (Smith 2010), two women with communication impairments who experienced initial difficulties in communicating with people not known to them described its impact on using services and recalling in similar terms counsellors who would try to second guess what they were saying. Helen described the frustration she felt during such occurrences:

> I would get quite uptight as it felt like the counsellor was trying to finish my sentences … to second guess what I was trying to say yet it was far removed from what I wanted to say and it felt like I was being rushed and the counsellor sometimes almost looked impatient … I think trying to second guess the counsellor thought they were being helpful but I just felt oppressed as it was like I couldn't express my own thoughts in my own time … the sessions being only an hour already bothered me but it was better for me to get a few things across that were my own thoughts and feelings rather than more stuff that wasn't actually what I wanted to say.
>
> Helen (age 41, congenital impairment)

Where communication difficulties exists, the importance of concentrating fully on what a client is conveying where non-verbal communication is being used in addition to the counsellor being honest about whether they have understood was emphasised by Wilson (2003). Attention was further drawn by Brearley and Bochley (1994) to how anxiety within a counsellor may block their ability to begin to work easily in an unfamiliar mode and that where recognised by the client this may potentially block their ability to use her or his system effectively. Additionally the need for counsellors to display sensitivity and to be flexible about the parameters of counselling sessions when working with disabled clients was stated by Olkin (1999), who drew attention to the potential of effects of impairment to impact on the frequency, timing and length of counselling sessions and is a topic that will be discussed within the next chapter.

Home Visits

A further factor of sensitive consideration within a counselling relationship and one which requires sensitive and careful judgement by the counsellor is that of home visits. Highlighted by the research data was how, for several women, counselling sessions within their own home would have been more convenient and practical than travelling to locations which regularly entailed considerable time and precious energy. Having received counselling on several occasions from a range of professionals and within a range of settings, Claire recalled her battles to have her need for home-based counselling recognised:

> Many times that I'd had counselling I'd gone along to the counsellors work base even though it was a huge effort physically and the travelling involved … getting motivated … it would have been much easier to have the sessions at home but I knew all the reasons why home visits weren't the norm … but on this one occasion I was mentally so low I knew I couldn't leave the house and physically I was really weak having not long had surgery and was still linked up to various medical bits so to travel to counselling just seemed impossible. The powers that be were quite adamant and said we could work around the health

> stuff but there was no understanding of the pain, energy, fatigue etc. Eventually my GP intervened and for a month I got visits at home which got me to a point where I then felt able to get to the counsellors work location … it was never about wanting special treatment it was about recognising individual need and that a one size fits all approach wasn't realistic.
>
> Claire (aged 39, acquired spinal illness)

In discussing the subject of home visits, Wilson (2003) acknowledged that for individuals with significant mobility impairments and/or physical health problems who are either seeking, or in need of professional counselling, leaving their home to meet in a neutral place may be difficult or for some impossible, and in such circumstances home visits are the only viable option. However, the lack of neutrality brought about by counselling taking place within the client's private space needs to be recognised alongside additional factors such as sharing of space, unexpected visitors or phone calls and the likelihood that providing therapeutic support within a client's home may be a compromise due to their home potentially containing varied memories and experiences that need to be addressed from a distance. Therefore, Wilson (2003) believes there to be a need for agreed boundaries between the counsellor and their client to be agreed so that the home environment can reflect as best as possible a counselling session taking place within a neutral space. However, whilst counselling literature overall does not favour home-based counselling by counsellors or hospital based psychologists and highlighting the importance of boundaries in maintaining the therapeutic frame (Clarkson 2003), likewise more recently, it has been argued (and particularly since the implementation of anti-discrimination legislation) that barriers can betray the counsellor if they fail to respond to the unique needs of an individual (Proctor 2008, Department of Health 2013). Evident from the study was a shared viewpoint in the need for professional guidelines to be balanced with individual needs and especially in the case of individuals for whom leaving home could have a detrimental impact on their physical and/or mental health, with an inability to leave the home not considered to be valid reasons for not providing the counselling support which an individual may require. In addition, Jack (2009) drew attention to disability legislation which now renders discrimination against disabled people to be unlawful and the legal obligations of counselling agencies and services in the early twenty-first century to now meet the access needs and requirements of people with physical (and visual and sensory) impairments and to ensure that reasonable adjustments are made.

Experiences of Mental Distress: Personal and Shared Viewpoints

Amongst the 12 women different forms of mental distress had been experienced and within Chapter 1 the diverse factors which women considered had contributed to those experiences and affected their mental well-being, for example, societal attitudes towards impairment or negative representations of disability were discussed. Additionally, whether the impairment was acquired or congenital in nature, experiences of mental distress were shown to have varied widely in their duration, frequency and severity. Having looked at both the issues of gender and impairment in addition to other factors which women considered to be of significance within the overall counselling process, the final part of the chapter will look at individual women's experiences of mental distress.

Bereavement and Mental Distress

Amongst the 12 women several had suffered a family bereavement or the loss of a significant person in their lives. Whilst women in the upper age ranges in particular recalled the scant availability of bereavement counselling in the mid-decades of the twentieth century, its wider availability today was felt to be indicative of a growing recognition of how bereavement can contribute to an onset of mental distress both for able-bodied and disabled women (and men). Born with her impairment, Katy believed the depression and episodes of feeling down which she had experienced over two decades had often been linked to the loss of her father, with whom she had a close relationship, when a young teenager, and a subsequent admission to residential care some months later was attributed with her becoming clinically depressed.

Similarly, the death of Elisabeth's husband from cancer in his mid-thirties was identified as having caused within her a deep sense of grief which developed into a depression and left her feeling unable to cope with everyday life, her depression exacerbated by a deep sense of anger felt towards medics who for many months dismissed Elisabeth's concerns about her husband's health:

> A few months after we married Charles became unwell and we were to and from the GP who insisted there was nothing wrong … I knew I was right but was dismissed as neurotic. By the time the cancer was found it was widespread and he died within a few weeks. Over time the anger built up as the outcome could have been different and combined with the grief I became very low and depressed … I agonised over whether I would have been listened to more if I'd been able-bodied and was convinced I would have been and just felt the doctor saw me as a disabled woman using her husband to get attention.
>
> Elisabeth (age 62, congenital impairment)

Physical Impairment and Mental Distress

For two women, the onset of depression was linked to their undergoing surgery related to their physical condition but which for both Carly and Philippa had only been partially successful in achieving its aims. Post-surgery, both women had endured prolonged pain and reduced mobility over several months which in turn had resulted in increased social isolation due in part to enforced extended absences from work which, for both women had provided a sense of normality and a structure to their lives. However, whilst the absence of paid work (which for some women also provided a sense of financial independence) and a daily structure to their lives was linked to experiences of mental distress for some women, for others the severity of their mental distress had led to a feeling of being unable to cope with the work environment. Recalling the effect of her mental distress on different aspects of her life, for many years Helen had perceived her mental distress to be more disabling than her physical impairment by virtue of her mental distress affecting both her body *and* her mind and at the height of her distress had felt unable to fulfil her commitments to either her paid or voluntary work due to an inability to function within either capacity. Mirrored sentiments were described by Alison who recalled the impact of her depression on her ability to work:

> When I was feeling down in myself after my marriage broke up I carried on at work as I needed something to focus on and to keep busy but as things got worse the depression was such that I couldn't get out of bed in the morning, couldn't brush my hair or brush my teeth … sort out clean clothes. All the stuff you just normally do automatically … it was all too much mentally and eventually I had to take time out from work until things were a lot better but the mental paralysis felt worse than the physical paralysis if that makes sense.
>
> Alison (age 38, congenital impairment)

Whilst, as previously discussed within Chapter 1 Helen (and other women) had considered their impairment to have been a contributory factor to their experiences of mental distress, Helen's diagnosis of breast cancer in her early thirties was also felt to have affected her mental health. A perceived unwillingness of other people to listen to the distress she was experiencing, in particularly in the months after diagnosis had been compounded by Helen's speech impairment and her difficulties in communicating verbally with others. Whilst recent advances in technology have enabled improved communication using a range of equipment, adapted technology and computer software, access to less advanced technology during the 1980s when experiencing acute distress had for Helen been limited with struggles to get appropriate support leaving her feeling effectively silenced:

> When I was diagnosed with breast cancer other women patients were offered counselling and whilst they talked about counselling for me it never happened and yet I was going through the same emotions as anyone else and was just as scared … I don't think they had treated a severely disabled patient with breast cancer before and nobody was quite sure what to do – it seemed like the two counsellors on the ward were both female as that was likely felt more appropriate and whilst my choice would always be as I've said to work with a male professional in this situation I would have given it a go but I just never got offered an opportunity … it was a lonely time.
>
> Helen (age 41, congenital impairment)

Having received an all-clear from her medical team after 18 months of treatment, for a short while Helen had attended a support group for women who had been successfully treated for breast cancer but who wished to informally meet within a forum where providing mutual support and sharing experiences was encouraged. Through the group Helen had learned how the issues covered within counselling sessions had typically been around the impact of breast cancer on self-image, in particular where a mastectomy had been necessary, and likewise the impact of diagnosis for women in personal relationships, both of which had led Helen to question whether this had been the reason for counselling not being offered to her:

> When I found this out and of course I can't know for sure but it did make me angry and quite upset as it made me think that their thoughts would be … oh well she will have poor self-image anyway because she's in a wheelchair … likewise they may have thought well it's unlikely Helen will be in a relationship so what's to be gained from offering her counselling … these would all have been assumptions I'm guessing made by medics who hardly knew me and regardless of whether I was a wheelchair-user or not … I was a patient with breast cancer like the other women on the ward and surely I should have had the same access to counselling as everyone else and I found it really hurtful.
>
> Helen (age 41, congenital impairment)

The highlighting of these and other factors served to reinforce the importance as discussed within Chapter 1 of mental health and allied professionals recognising that whilst an individual's physical impairment may be a contributory factor within the overall experience of mental distress, it may not always be the case and the vital need to give much greater consideration to a range of factors or circumstances that may have the potential to impact on mental well-being was called for group-wide.

Other Aspects of Mental Distress

Diagnosed with Multiple Sclerosis in her early thirties, Maria described how one of her greatest difficulties following her diagnosis had been in dealing with the sadness she experienced linked to health difficulties being endured by one of her children. The nature and extent of her condition had left Maria feeling unable to provide the support her child needed and she believed herself not to be fulfilling her role as a mother:

> Whilst I struggled to come to terms with the MS diagnosis I'd had to be strong and be there for my family yet a lot of my upset was about when the children as teenagers and one especially were having problems yet I felt I couldn't provide them with the support they needed because of my all round limitations … they knew I loved them and told them all the time even when my speech became affected and I couldn't physically put my arms around them to give them a big

> hug which was upsetting … they could do that to me which was lovely and I needed that but as their mum I wanted to hold them, hug them and tell them things would be ok even though there were no guarantees.
>
> Maria (age 51, acquired neurological impairment)

Having lived with her acquired impairment for almost three decades, Jackie recalled how in the initial weeks after sustaining her injury she retreated into herself but that the support provided by family, friends and fellow patients on the spinal unit had encouraged her to remain positive and to adapt to living a 'normal' life but in a different way. In contrast, Claire's first experience of acute mental distress had not occurred until four years after the onset of her impairment when the reality dawned that it was to be a permanent feature of her life, recalling how until then she had naively considered herself to be 'different' and believing she would regain her able-bodied status. Both women considered the young age at which they acquired their impairments to have been significant to their first experiences of mental distress occurring some time after acquiring their impairments, each believing that their young age would offer protection from a permanently disabled status but that this false belief was not recognised until some years after onset of impairment. Additionally, both women commented that having just entered adolescence when their respective impairments were acquired, neither had been in relationships nor following chosen career paths, both of which were factors which women who acquired their impairments as adults considered to be linked to their experiences of mental distress. Therefore, both Jackie and Claire held a shared view that although adapting to their impairment had been both physically and mentally challenging, their youth had enabled them to 'restart' their lives but within a new set of parameters.

Over the three decades spent living with her acquired impairment Claire had experienced numerous prolonged episodes of mental distress many of which had required treatment from both community and hospital based mental health professionals. During episodes of acute mental distress Claire had often seriously self-harmed with superficial self-harming having routinely been used as a coping mechanism to help release feelings of angst during times of distress. Two attempted suicides, both of which had warranted hospital admission and additional periodic episodes of acute distress combined with enduring eating distress, Claire recalled as having led to her becoming identified by her mental health conditions and expressed dissatisfaction at the way in which 'labels' had become attached to her. In particular, Claire recalled her difficulty in accepting a diagnosis of Anorexia Nervosa, believing the onset of her eating distress to have originated from a sense of loss felt both for what she had experienced during her teenage years and for the opportunities she considered had been denied her as a consequence of becoming severely paralysed when barely a teenager:

> It just increasingly felt like I had no control over anything … decisions being made all around you and for you yet not with you … like you had stopped being a real

> person … my food intake seemed to be the one thing I could control independently – for everything else I just seemed to have become some symbol of dependency as I needed help with pretty much everything and it was really tough.
>
> Claire (age 39, acquired spinal illness)

The experience of eating distress during her teenage years Claire described as being the starting point for problems with food intake over many years but with which she had learned to live, and that with the long-term support of friends now considered herself to be 'sensible' about her food intake. Whilst a full 'recovery' or a return to 'normal' eating patterns was felt to be unlikely, Claire had felt proud that for over a decade she had been in control of her eating habits as opposed to the food controlling her and taking up her every waking thought. Of her suicide attempts, Claire recalled how difficult and intensive counselling sessions with a psychologist had enabled her to recognise that both attempts had resulted from feeling unable to cope any longer with her life in its then present state. In the weeks preceding her suicide attempts Claire spoke of her unsuccessful efforts to get mental health nurses to listen to the distress she was experiencing but that her distressing thoughts had escalated to a point at which she had acted upon them and subsequently was admitted to acute psychiatric care.

Stigma and Mental Distress

As the eldest participant, Elisabeth described how during episodes of acute distress, which were primarily linked to experiencing a decline in her physical abilities, she had felt 'on the edge of going mad'. An inability to verbally express how she was feeling Elisabeth attributed to her perception of a continuing stigma through the mid-decades of the twentieth century to be suffering from mental illness with support for her views reaffirmed by data which evidenced the efforts made, in particular by women aged over 50 to conceal their mental distress from others. A real sense of reluctance to share with husbands, partners, family or significant people in their lives that they were experiencing (or had experienced) mental distress and were receiving treatment/support was voiced by a number of women with Maria keen to refer to her distress as 'sadness' or 'a down time' rather than the depression which in reality she knew it to be. Recalling their experiences of living with depression, several women shared the view that whilst generally people no longer referred to hospitals for the treatment of people with mental illness as 'asylums', and that people were now seldom referred to as 'insane' or 'mad'. However, there remained a belief across the group that until latter decades of the twentieth century, within society people had broadly continued to equate people diagnosed with depression or other mental health conditions as being 'mentally ill' alongside a perception that people would be treated in long stay institutions that were sheltered from public view. Thus, like other women Maria had been anxious of becoming labelled as 'mad' or 'mentally ill';

> When during the nineties I tried to get counselling I felt there had been a slight shift in attitudes towards mental ill health though I still felt a bit ashamed and embarrassed about asking and even today I'd be less likely to talk openly about being depressed than if say I'd broken my arm. Physical ill health is more tangible, often visual and understood in a way that mental ill health has never historically been … people still remember the old locked wards and people thinking that people in those places were mad …
>
> Maria (age 51, acquired neurological impairment)

However, evident from the study was the shared belief that the historical stigma attached to mental illness had to some extent in more recent decades gradually lessened and showing a broad consensus that within society people now talk more openly about feeling depressed or as experiencing some form of mental or psychological distress for example, stress or anxiety though it was also considered that women were more likely to talk about their mental health than men. In the government survey Attitudes to Mental Illness (2011) public attitudes towards mental health were shown to be becoming less discriminatory; of 1,741 people surveyed, 77 per cent agreed with the written statement given 'that mental illness is an illness like any other illness' compared with a figure of 71 per cent 15 years previously whilst the percentage of people who stated they would feel comfortable talking to a friend or family about their mental health issues increased from 66 per cent in 2009 to 70 per cent in 2011.

Furthermore, women considered there to now exist within twenty-first-century society a better awareness around more recognised mental health conditions for example, depression, stress and anxiety, but that unequivocally there remained scope for a much greater improvement of understanding, awareness and acceptance of mental ill health within society at large and in particular by work employers. Recent years have seen a number of campaigns led by mental health organisations or charities in conjunction with government departments which have received coverage within national newspapers, television, radio and on advertising billboards and featuring people with personal experience of mental distress such campaigns have aimed to both raise awareness of mental ill health and to eradicate stigma and discrimination. Founded in 2007 (and currently funded until 2015) and led by mental health charities Mind and Rethink Mental Illness, *Time to Change* is England's biggest ever programme designed to tackle stigma and discrimination. Whilst *It's Time to Talk* (Mind 2012) aimed to tackle the fear and awkwardness that people feel around talking about mental health. More recently, Mind's campaign, *It's the Little Things* (Mind 2014) presents the small things that people can do to support someone experiencing mental health problems such as having a cup of tea with someone or making a phone call to talk to an individual affected.

Conclusions

This chapter sought firstly to examine the significance of gender within the counselling process and to consider the reasoning for the preferences that were expressed across the sample group to work with a female or male counsellor. Secondly, it likewise wished to examine expressed preferences to work with a counsellor with lived experience of impairment (or someone who by virtue of their personal circumstances had a good understanding and awareness of issues around disability and impairment) or alternatively a non-disabled counsellor. Whilst the large majority of women's preference to work with a female counsellor had been based on a shared perception that a female would have a better understanding of their mental distress, in particular if their distress was linked to gender or gender roles, that a counsellor of gender choice could not provide an automatic guarantee of a positive counselling experience was shown to be acknowledged. Other attributes or factors such as a counsellors personality, character traits or their socio-economic background were all recognised to potentially, singularly or combined, be of significance. Furthermore, a counsellor's ability to communicate effectively with, and to listen to what their client was saying were all considered to have the ability to impact on whether the counselling experience was rated positively or otherwise.

Just as the chapter has shown there to be no definitive answer as to whether disabled women would have a more positive counselling experience if the counsellor worked with was of the same gender, likewise the chapter has indicated there to be no clear evidence of whether people with a physical impairment benefit from receiving counsellors who have lived experience of impairment, or by virtue of for example, being a long-term carer for a disabled person may have a good understanding and awareness of disability and impairment related issues. Preferences to work with a counsellor with personal experience of impairment had been based on a belief that such individuals would have a good understanding of their mental distress by virtue of their own circumstances, whilst others emphasised the importance of recognising that no two people will live with, or experience their impairment in an identical way. A wish to work with a non-disabled counsellor, it has been suggested may have resulted from internalised oppression, with the disabled individual feeling that a disabled counsellor will not be 'as good' as an able-bodied counsellor, whilst the view that a disabled counsellor was not necessary if the issues relating to the client's mental distress were not linked to their physical impairment per se was shared by some women.

Whilst the chapter has considered the possible advantages or otherwise of working with a disabled counsellor, group-wide women were not in favour of disabled clients only being counselled by disabled counsellors, believing this could potentially lead over time to a return of the segregation of able-bodied and disabled people that had historically been commonplace until the mid-twentieth century. However, whilst preferences to work with a disabled counsellor were expressed both within my work and that of others (Reeve 2008, Jack 2009), the research findings demonstrated clearly that choice had been available only in exceptional circumstances, or for those who self-funded their counselling. Whilst the expansion of counselling in the UK over recent decades has led to an increase in the number of available able-bodied counsellors (and trainee counsellors) this has failed to be matched by a growth in the number of disabled counsellors available, thus resulting in the call for greater opportunities for disabled people who wish to train as counsellors. Allowing more flexibility in admission criteria to professional training courses whilst maintaining professional standards it was believed would enable a greater consideration of an individual's life experiences and circumstances and what they could bring to a counselling relationship. Until this occurred, disabled people who wished to work with a disabled counsellor, it was believed would neither have their voices heard nor their wishes granted. An increased presence of disabled trainees within the classroom, combined with a greater focus on disability and impairment within course syllabuses, it was further hoped could slowly but steadily reverse the current lack of counsellors UK-wide who specialise in working with disabled clients. These changes, alongside others which, based on their personal experiences of mental distress and working with mental health professionals, women believed needed to take place will now be examined within Chapter 5.

Chapter 5
Future Mental Health Provision: A Need for Change?

Introduction

Previous chapters have shown how women's experiences of receiving effective and appropriate mental health support had been affected by a widely shared perception that a significant proportion of the mental health professionals with whom they had worked had little awareness or understanding of issues relating to physical impairment and/or disability. In addition, most professionals had little knowledge of the rights of disabled people under the Disability Discrimination Act and had been unfamiliar with either social model approaches to disability or using social model approaches within their work with disabled clients. Within this chapter, the consideration of factors such as the inclusion of disability equality training, teaching around the social model of disability and its principles, and an element of service-user involvement within the professional training courses of counsellors and other mental health and social care professionals working with disabled people both within the context of providing support, and the approaches used by professionals when working with disabled women (and men) will be discussed.

Secondly, the chapter will examine the study's findings relating to how disability legislation over recent decades, in particular the implementation of the Disability Discrimination Act (1995) was believed to have impacted on women's mental well-being. Additionally, it will discuss the perceived need for mental health professionals to have a greater awareness of how the problematic representation of disability within the media can affect in diverse ways the mental well-being of disabled women (and men).

Finally, in revisiting the structural and organisational barriers that women encountered in gaining access to, and using mental health services which were examined within Chapter 2, the changes which women considered needed to happen in aiming to provide in the years ahead, improved, effective and appropriate mental health services for disabled women who experience mental distress will be discussed.

Training of Mental Health Professionals

Based on personal experiences of using mental health services and working with mental health professionals across a range of services and organisations, analysed interview and focus group data highlighted a number of ways in which women considered that the future training of counsellors, psychologists and other mental health professionals throughout the UK could be improved. Both the inclusion of disability equality training and teaching around the social model of disability within courses syllabuses were changes which along with others were suggested and each of which will now be considered below.

Disability Equality Training

One of the consistent themes to emerge from the study, and discussed in previous chapters was the overwhelming need for all mental health professionals who work with disabled women (and men) to gain a greater knowledge, understanding and awareness of disability and impairment if future mental health provision is to meet effectively and appropriately the mental health needs of disabled women who experience mental distress. Through changes being made to the training courses of counsellors, psychologists and relevant professionals, women believed this could be achieved with the perceived need for disability equality training to be routinely incorporated into the syllabus of professional training courses repeatedly asserted across the sample group.

Developed by disabled people in the late 1980s to address the need for improved and accurate information about disability, disability equality training (DET) aims to assist people in gaining a greater understanding of the meaning of disability with the need for DET to be included within counselling training asserted by Lago and Smith (2004). A recurrent theme within the study was the need for counsellors and allied professionals to address their own attitudes to disability so that they neither patronise or oppress disabled clients further by colluding with the traditional social norm of trying to 'rescue' or keep disabled people as dependent, and maintaining an adherence to loss theories with each being areas which women believed there to be scope within professional training courses to address. Through including DET within courses syllabuses, women considered that the professionals of tomorrow would be provided with opportunities to address any such thoughts, feelings and attitudes towards disability and/or impairment and would aim to ensure that any conscious or unconscious prejudices they may have do not contaminate the therapeutic relationship with disabled clients. In addition, the opportunity for counsellors (or other professionals who may provide counselling as part of their work role with disabled clients) to discuss within counselling any prejudices or discomfort they may hold in relation to intimate or sexual issues was considered to be imperative (Shakespeare 2000, Crawford and Ostrove 2003) so that disabled clients are not denied the opportunity to discuss such matters if they so choose (Bonnie 2004). Within my own research (Smith 2010) and that of Jack (2009) some participants had felt judged by their counsellor when they had endeavoured to explore any personal sexual frustrations or difficulties and that any discussion had been blocked by the counsellor's visible discomfort. A need to talk about sexual issues Jack (2009) believed to reflect the view of a wider social population, highlighting a study undertaken by a UK-wide disability publication of 1,115 people of both sexes with a diagnosed physical impairment (Disability Now 2005). Within the study 93.6 per cent were shown to have nobody to confide in about sexual matters and had low sexual self-esteem compared with 68.2 per cent amongst those who had someone available in whom they could confide. Whilst 68 per cent of the survey group stipulated a need for a specialist psycho-sexual counselling service for disabled people, the reality is that mainstream counselling services are likely to be the only option available to disabled clients within the statutory sector.

Through the future widespread provision of DET within UK training courses of counsellors and other mental health professionals who may work with disabled clients, women hoped that mental health professionals would find ways to challenge the organisational behaviours which traditionally have reinforced negative myths and values about disabled people and which have prevented individuals from gaining equality and achieving full participation in society. Therefore, until DET was mandatorily included within professional training courses (and with a requirement for professionals to attend any updated training as was deemed helpful or necessary), professionals currently practising with little knowledge of, and/or a lack of awareness or understanding of disability and impairment, it was felt would continue to work in ways which were deemed to provide little benefit to disabled people in need of effective mental health intervention or support. Likewise, the undertaking of further research within the arguably under examined topic area of physical impairment and mental distress, Jack (2009) believed would assist in ascertaining whether the inclusion of DET, which she considered to be a desirable addition to core training curriculums, needs to be considered by the British Association for Counselling and Psychotherapy.

The Social Model of Disability

In signalling a radical shift in thinking about disability in the latter decades of the twentieth century, the social model of disability recast disability as a form of social oppression and threw a spotlight on the need for societal change and the removal of socially created barriers and all forms of institutional discrimination which had dominated for many decades. Within the social model 'impairment' is defined as 'functional limitations which affect a person's body' whilst 'disability' is defined as 'loss or limitations of opportunities arising from direct and indirect discrimination'. Developed out of the need of growing numbers of disabled people in the UK wanting to challenge discrimination against them and to assert their rights to accessible services, employment and full participation in social activities, the rise of the social model came to question the idea that an individual was responsible for the 'tragedy' of their disability. Likewise, a medical model approach in which individuals had historically been defined and constricted by a medical diagnosis and often imposed upon disabled people by medical or health professionals, came to be increasingly challenged and rejected. In contrast to the medical model of disability, the social model of disability (SMOD) shifts the focus from impairment onto disability, locating disability neither within an impaired or malfunctioning body (Marks 1999) but within an excluding and oppressive social environment and reinforcing how many restrictions imposed on disabled people have long been a product of an environment which failed to take account of their needs as opposed to being a natural or inevitable consequence of their impairment (Oliver 1990).

Clearly evidenced by the study data was a belief that whilst mental health professionals continued to work within a medical model approach to disability in which women were characterised by what they were *un*able to do, and working with the assumption that the woman's impairment was the primary reason for their mental distress, that women would continue to receive inappropriate support which was ineffective and which would did not meet their needs. Conversely, by professionals becoming familiar with, and adopting a social model approach to disability within their work with disabled clients, women believed would lead to increased positive reporting of receiving mental health support that had proved valuable in addressing their mental distress. Furthermore, a good knowledge of the social model of disability, it was believed, would enable a greater understanding of the way in which disabled people may often internalise oppression and was deemed important for therapists to be aware of.

The marked improvements in the lives of disabled people since the latter decades of the twentieth century which, to a significant degree have resulted from the challenges made to structural disablism and the introduction of anti-discrimination legislation, have been acknowledged by both academics and disabled people (Smith 2003, Oliver 2004, Pring 2008). However, an emphasis on the barriers 'out there' Thomas (1999) claimed has resulted in the ironic consequences of leaving aspects of social life and social oppression which are so keenly felt by many disabled people (to do with self-esteem and image etc.), open season to psychologists and others who would not hesitate to apply the personal tragedy model to these issues.

In seeking for an extension of the social model of disability, which focused not just on the removal of structural barriers but which was also concerned for 'who we are prevented from being' and how we feel and think about ourselves, Thomas (1999) claimed would thus facilitate a sophisticated analysis of the manner in which disabled people (women and men) are disabled by oppressive social relations. For many disabled people, Reeve (2008) claims it to be the barriers that operate within oneself at the psycho emotional level which have the most disabling effects on their lives and that it is time for this dimension of disablism which operates along both emotional and psychological pathways to be given proper attention within disability theory and within disability practice (Smith 2010, Reeve 2012, 2013). Whilst such experiences have been shown to create feelings of anger and rejection for disabled people, the psychological consequences are only just belatedly beginning to be considered in earnest.

Service-user Involvement

In seeking to improve future mental health provision across the UK for women, Connor and Wilson (2006) commented on the importance of mental health professionals learning from service-users both about their personal experiences of mental distress and of receiving mental health support. In striving to gain a broader understanding and awareness of issues relating to disability and impairment, the introduction of service-user input to counselling and mental health training courses was identified as another way in which the training of mental health professionals who upon qualification may work with disabled clients could be improved in the years ahead. Through listening to the personal stories of individuals with lived-experience of both physical impairment and mental distress, women believed that professionals who may play a key role in supporting disabled clients who are experiencing mental distress could improve their overall understanding and awareness of disability and impairment, in addition to learning from lecture based teaching and books. Group-wide there existed a consensus that both health and mental health professionals were cautious of learning from service-users due to a wariness of considering unfamiliar methods within their professional training and may feel that as 'professionals' (or trainee professionals) they know best and that it is *us*, (disabled people) who need *their* (mental health/health professionals) help, knowledge and expertise. However, group-wide women believed there to be no substitute for personal experience and that whilst well-meaning individuals may endeavour to empathise with someone living with a physical impairment, a true and full understanding could only come from lived personal experience. Alison stated:

> I think these so called professionals need to listen to what we are saying rather than just assuming they know what is best which is how things have worked for so long ... it's not everyone but for many people I think there's a feeling of well we have the qualifications so we are the experts ... you're the people we are here to help. But I really feel that professionals and trainees need to learn from real people as well as books and from sitting in the classroom ... we've had the lived-experience so please listen to how we felt going through mental distress ... learn from us.
>
> Alison (age 38, congenital impairment)

Group-wide, as the health professional who for the majority of women had been the first point of contact when seeking mental health support, GPs were identified as one group of health professionals who needed to develop a greater understanding of disability and impairment, yet disappointingly were considered unlikely to give to support service-user initiatives. As a patient representative who for a number of years had spoken to local health groups, Lisa recalled GPs' routine absences:

> Each time I gave a talk the local GPs would be invited alongside other health and social care professionals but overwhelmingly it was the doctors who didn't

> show up generally saying they were too busy. Personally I think it was more to do with a lack of interest and a feeling they wouldn't learn anything from us as service-users … also I think most doctors don't really see physical disability or mental health as particularly exciting areas of medicine. I may be wrong but it's what my experiences have led me to believe.
>
> Lisa (age 45, congenital impairment)

Since the latter years of the twentieth century a growing number of academic institutions offering training courses/degrees within social care for example, Social Work degree courses have included within their syllabuses or curriculum an element of service-user input in which people, who have had contact with social care organisations/professionals, including people with physical impairments (or carers of) or mental health survivors are involved within elements of trainees' professional training for example, assessing students fitness to practise through role play scenarios and talking to trainees about their personal experiences of working with social workers or other social care professionals. Having made a service-user contribution to the undergraduate social work degree course at her local university for nine years, Jackie had found the experience to be positive at a number of levels:

> Having firstly attended some training the university offered it was really interesting to get involved in the interviews of people who were applying to study social work … you could look back on your own experiences of working with social workers and think oh yes this person would have been great or otherwise and it was interesting to see how course selectors chose people … But getting involved either on your own or with others in the teaching input to courses and sharing your personal experiences that has been brilliant … people are listening to your experiences but more than that they are learning from it and every year the student evaluations show how much the students find the service-user input a positive experience and I think the same would bring great benefits for mental health professionals, for them and their clients.
>
> Jackie (age 45, congenital impairment)

With government policies now developed in such a way that statutory authorities are required to consult with disabled people (and other minimised groups), the Health and Social Care Act 2011 (Department of Health 2012) places a duty on NHS organisations to involve patients both in the planning and development of service provision and in decisions affecting operations of those services, women felt there was much to be gained from increased service-user input within the training courses of mental health professionals. Through increasing counsellors and allied professionals knowledge base, understanding and awareness of impairment, women believed service-user input would in turn help to improve disabled people's experiences of receiving mental health support.

Evidenced by the study and commented upon previously, was how a counsellor's lack of knowledge about disability had been a barrier to effective therapy taking place. Three women described in similar terms how they had found themselves to be playing the role of an educator and that this was felt to add weight to the potential benefits of service-user involvement within the training courses of mental health professionals. Furthermore, the incorporation of service-user involvement within training courses women believed would be beneficial in that in addition to trainees being given the opportunity to learn about individual's lived experiences of impairment and mental distress, trainee professionals would be enabled to gain a greater understanding of individual's reasoning for other suggested organisational and practical changes which were considered needed to happen in striving to improve future mental health provision. These factors will now be considered.

Impairment-related Factors: A Need for Consideration

Further evidenced by the study was the need for mental health professionals to gain through their training a greater awareness of the practical issues linked to their impairment that a disabled person may have to consider, and that future experiences of using mental health services could be improved considerably through professionals displaying a greater appreciation of an individual's specific circumstances and/or needs. Additionally highlighted was the real need for all counsellors and mental health professionals working with disabled clients to display sensitivity and flexibility around the parameters of counselling sessions alongside a recognition of the possible effects of an individual's impairment on the frequency, time of day and length of counselling sessions; whilst, for example, a counselling session of an hour's duration may for some individuals be too long due to pain or discomfort, conversely for someone with a communication impairment additional time may be welcomed (Jack 2009). Further, a greater consideration of both the suitability and accessibility of the service location was called for, in particular by women with severely impaired mobility who further emphasised the need for better awareness among mental health professionals working with disabled clients of issues such as the availability of accessible transport and/or care assistance which may affect when, or if appointment times can be met. A failure to give due consideration to her speech impairment when receiving counselling was described by Helen:

> When I was having my counselling sessions through the NHS I was told the sessions would be 50 minutes minimum but not exceeding an hour. Well because of my speech I could hardly talk about anything in that length of time yet there was no flexibility or thought given to my specific circumstances … it was so frustrating and all the effort of getting there hardly seemed worthwhile.
>
> Helen, (age 41, congenital impairment)

As discussed within Chapter 1 several women recalled their experiences of mental distress as having been linked to factors other than their impairment per se. For some women, the provision of personal and practical care support from private agencies had often been experienced as ad hoc and numerous examples of the care provider's inflexibility in accommodating their often changing needs and requirements were cited. Women described having to explain to the mental health professionals with whom they were working, the ways in which the structure of their daily live could often be determined by their care needs and likewise their potential to impact on mental and psychological wellbeing. The need for improved training which includes reference to psycho-emotional disablism Reeve (2008) believes has the potential to play an important role in the move to professionals providing care that is both supportive and enabling. Likewise, the need for training that also includes a focus on practical considerations and individual needs was supported group-wide and that until counsellors and allied professionals were able to provide support that recognised each of these aspects then disabled women (and men) would continue to receive services which were not tailored to their needs and that a one-size-fits-all approach would continue unchallenged.

The Disability Discrimination Act and its Impact on Mental Well-being

In seeking to determine whether there existed a causal link between improved environmental access and positive mental well-being the study provided evidence of a shared belief that the legislative changes which had expanded throughout the 1980s (the Disabled Persons Act 1981 sought to address access and adaptation of building issues for people with mobility difficulties, the Disabled Persons Act 1986 further sought to legislate and improve control over services provided for their use and following years of striving for anti-discrimination legislation 1995 finally welcomed the introduction of the DDA) had been a major development both in terms of the substantially improved access to the environment, buildings and services and in having a positive effect on women's mental and psychological well-being. Moving into a new millennium, analysed data showed a broadly shared belief in disability awareness within society being higher than ever before with opportunities now available for disabled people (though some considered not all) to break away from some of the confined roles and opportunities which had historically been ascribed to them. A report from the Prime Minister's strategy unit, 'Improving the Life Chances of Disabled People' was significant in emphasising the need for disabled people to have greater control over their lives and endorsed explicitly for the first time the social model of disability:

> Disability is the disadvantage that comes from barriers which impact on people with impairments.
>
> PMSU 2005

The DDA (2005) further widened the remit of discrimination by increasing the number of organisations and services that were required to ensure non-discrimination against disabled people whilst also placing a duty on every local authority to promote equality of opportunity (Fillingham 2012). Currently, the Equality Act (2010) in aiming to strengthen, simplify and harmonise seven existing pieces of legislation including the DDA now provides a framework which is intended to protect the rights of individuals and to achieve equality of opportunity for all.

Whilst the witnessed improvements in structural accessibility had been welcomed group-wide, they were considered to have been long overdue with feelings of anger and frustration expressed that it had taken until the early twenty-first century to attain the level of access to the environment that disabled people now had and that undoubtedly scope for further improvement remained. Likewise, the slow pace at which changes had happened, had for most women created a feeling of being 'less important' than able-bodied people alongside a sense of feeling like second-class citizens with many small shop owners and businesses considered to have been slow and/or unwilling to make the necessary changes to make their premises accessible, having used loopholes within the legislation to avoid the costs associated with any required modifications. Marks (1999) claimed that many attempts to overcome physical and social barriers have been only partially successful; Barnes (2010) further drew attention to the progress that still needs to be made in becoming a society in which disabled people are fully included. For example, many disabled toilets continue to be combined with baby changing facilities or alternatively may be used for storage of cleaning materials in addition to sometimes being poorly designed. Reeve (2008) has similarly drawn attention to scenarios in which disabled people, most likely wheelchair-users may still be expected to enter shops through makeshift rear entrances or in which upper shop levels can only be accessed through use of goods or services lifts and none of which would be expected of, nor would be acceptable to able-bodied customers.

Alison described her total avoidance of a shop in her local town due to the negative messages which she perceived the shop owner to be giving to disabled customers:

> There's a little gift shop that people say sells nice little things but it has a notice on the shop front window saying 'if you need help please knock on the window … how humiliating … one day the shop owner came out and said they could bring anything out if I knew what I wanted but I'd just wanted to browse like any other customer. It was all the more frustrating as it's only a small step and they could quite easily get a ramp.
>
> Alison (age 38, congenital impairment)

Likewise, Lisa spoke with angst about a bold print notice pinned to the window of her local coffee shop:

> The notice in the window says 'due to limited space, please no prams, pushchairs or walking frames' … I'm sure they'd like to have included wheelchairs within that but know they can't get away with it and the message is just so unwelcoming in this day and age I think it would put me off even if I wasn't disabled.
>
> Lisa (age 45, congenital impairment)

Several women recalled experiences of difficulties in accessing shops or public places yet were frustrated by them still seemingly meeting the 'reasonable adjustments' legally required of them. However, even where access requirements had been met at a structural level, attention was drawn by three women, each a wheelchair-user who continued to feel that full equal access was to yet become a reality. With views supported by fellow participants, Philippa described how her visits to local theatres and cinemas continued to differ from those of her able-bodied friends:

> Whilst I'm really pleased that as someone who loves film and theatre I can now get into different theatres and cinemas in the area around me I still get annoyed that I have to sit in a certain place where they have chosen as opposed to being able to choose where I would like to sit … and of course the often reduced rates for seats are welcome but the fact you can only have one companion or carer sit alongside you annoys me as I have a big circle of friends and we go out as a group yet you get to the film or show and have to be separated so I think there's still work to do.
>
> Philippa (age 36, congenital impairment)

Similarly, Carly spoke of her frustration that despite being able to exit buildings such as cinemas independently in her powered wheelchair, entry was often only permitted if she was accompanied by an able-bodied person:

> It does annoy me as I'm an adult and in the unlikely event of a fire I could get out as quick if not quicker than other people using my full speed control yet unlike an able-bodied person I can't see a show or film on my own … if I let it, it can get me down as underneath its still sending a message I feel that as someone in a wheelchair you're different and mentally it can affect you but I try to remember the progress that's been made.
>
> Carly (age 18, congenital impairment)

Access to Public Transport

Likewise, women acknowledged the progress made in recent decades in making public transport accessible to disabled people and in particular to wheelchair-users who historically had been unable to access buses, trains etc. and which was widely welcomed. The improvements had been key for those without access to private transport in enabling access to public places from which they hitherto had largely been excluded (Prideaux 2006). However, a shared belief in the need for more progress to be made UK-wide in making all forms of public transport fully accessible to people with physical (and other forms of) impairments was emphasised in particular by women living in rural or semi-rural locations where transport links were less integrated and for those unable to afford privately owned transport due to their often considerable cost (Lawson and Matthews 2005). Alison described the barriers she had encountered in accessing suitable transport:

> Where I live is quite rural and there are only a couple of buses to the village each day and growing up they were never accessible for my wheelchair and still aren't … mum and dad had a car but putting the wheelchair in and out of the car and lifting me in and out of the car for years wasn't ideal especially I was growing up … it used to frustrate me that once you got to the mainline rail station with the help of staff you could get pretty much anywhere in the UK even though for many years travelling in the guards van was hardly a dignified experience. I learned to drive as soon as I was able to but then had to save for an adapted car which is my lifeline now but with the high costs involved keeping it on the road it can feel like a luxury and I now use it really just when I need to.
>
> Alison (age 38, congenital impairment)

Mental Well-being

In addition to the recognised ways in which improved access to buildings, spaces and public transport had helped women at a structural level, evidenced by the data was how the structural changes had also impacted positively on mental well-being with Jackie having commented, for example:

> When the building I'd been working in for years finally got a lift installed it made such a difference to my working day … for years I'd had to trudge around the outside of the building in all weathers to access it at the level where I worked which got to be tiring and took energy I really needed for my working day … But more than that it meant I went into the building the same way as everyone else and daft as it sounds it gave me a mental boost because it made me feel an equal … gave me a sense of normality.
>
> Jackie, (age 45, acquired spinal cord injury)

Elisabeth also spoke of how the environmental changes had brought greater opportunities to engage in activities which she had previously been denied access to. This in turn had provided the mental stimulation she had long sought unsuccessfully, with her newly acquired ability to access social arenas having enabled increased social contact with able-bodied and disabled people alike. Furthermore, in assisting in forging friendships, Elisabeth recalled long-held feelings of social isolation slowly beginning to diminish which simultaneously had a positive effect on her overall mental health and well-being.

Disability Representation in the Media and Self-image

Clearly demonstrated by the research evidence and commented upon in Chapter 1, was the importance that women attached to having a positive self-image and that 'looking presentable' or 'dressing nicely' had helped women to feel 'normal' whilst also providing a confidence boost and improving to varying degrees, overall feelings of self-worth. However, evidenced clearly by the data was the group-wide consensus of the substantial role played by the UK media in affecting, overwhelmingly in a negative way, the self-image of disabled women and that over many decades, across television, film, magazines or written material, there had persistently been minimal real or accurate representation of how the majority of disabled women live their daily lives. In particular, attention was drawn by Finkelstein (1987) and Marks (1999) to how the portrayal of physical (and other forms of) impairment on television has long failed to reflect the statistical incidence of impairment within wider society. This was claimed to be especially true within soap operas which in traditionally meaning to represent everyday life within a range of UK communities had, with minority exceptions, i.e. Sandy played a wheelchair-user character in *Crossroads* during the 1970s, failed to cast characters with any form of physical impairment. Whilst during the latter stages of the twentieth century disabled people or characters began to be seen on television screens, overwhelmingly they were cast in programmes where the content has been disability related, for example, hate crime, euthanasia, welfare benefits, government cuts to services etc. whilst disabled characters within series dramas or soap operas were played by non-disabled actors, for example, Chris King as a wheelchair-user in *Emmerdale* and Maud Grimes as a powered-wheelchair-user in *Coronation Street.*

However, evident from the study was that moving into a new millennium, women believed that progress had been made on a number of levels and was continuing to be made in relation to a slowly improving representation of disability across different media forms, in particular within television, and which in turn was considered to be playing a role in improving women's self-image. This belief was mirrored by Reeve (2008) who drew attention to the importance of positive images of disabled people in the media and a growing disability arts movement, neither of which she felt could be understated in helping people move towards a more positive position. A greater presence of disabled people across a range of television programmes, for example, within news programmes, BBC War Correspondent Frank Gardner, wheelchair-user contestants on daytime game shows, a teenage comedian with cerebral palsy as a finalist on *Britain's Got Talent* in 2013 and a wheelchair-user actor in *Coronation Street*. In addition soap storylines have been both applauded and criticised for tackling sensitive issues sometimes associated with progressive or long-term disabilities such as euthanasia (*Emmerdale* 2012) and ending one's own life (*Coronation Street* 2013) but which for large numbers of disabled people was welcomed for bringing to the fore topics which are often steered away from. Furthermore, recent years have seen on television screens programmes in which disabled people have been the main focus, including *Britain's Top Disabled Model*, which was considered by some to have given young disabled women an opportunity to pursue their chosen career whilst criticised by others for its segregation of disabled and non-disabled women. Likewise, whilst supporters of *The Undateables* (Channel 4 2013, 2014) believed the programme to sensitively publicise the difficulties or prejudices that disabled people may encounter in seeking personal relationships, critics felt that the programmes title immediately presented physical impairment in a negative light, in particular within the context of seeking a relationship and was felt to ridicule some aspects of disabled people's health conditions.

In receiving extensive media and television coverage, the London Paralympics 2012 was, across society, considered to have positively influenced the attitudes of able-bodied people towards disabled people and disability per se and not just their abilities to compete and achieve in sport at a professional level. In addition, the then government spoke of the Paralympics as having provided new and more opportunities for disabled people to participate in society both in sport and in other areas. However, whilst the success of the Paralympics and the participating Paralympians resulted in a positive shift in attitudes towards both disabled people and disability itself, questions began to be raised among disability organisations as to the long-term benefits. To mark the first anniversary of the Paralympics, Scope (2013) conducted a survey using social media to seek the views of disabled people as to whether the event had impacted on their lives and disappointingly found the legacy of the Paralympics to be hanging in the balance with disabled people remaining concerned about public attitudes to disability. Of the 1,015 people interviewed, 8 per cent felt that attitudes towards them had not improved in the year since the Paralympics had ended whilst 22 per cent believed attitudes had worsened and amongst whom 84 per cent felt that recent media coverage of benefit claims and the welfare system had had a negative effect on public attitudes towards disabled people.

Further evidenced by the study findings was women's widespread dissatisfaction of the ways in which disabled women (and men) are commonly portrayed in the media either as heroes, courageous individuals, charitable cases or victims who should be pitied and offered sympathy. Likewise, the frequent portrayal of disabled people as tragic victims (in particular disabled children) which have long been a staple of charity advertising and fund raising that has relied on evoking feelings of pity, in turn pulling on the heartstrings of able-bodied people in the hope they will be sufficiently 'moved' to make a financial donation (and making themselves feel better in the process) were objected to. Recent decades however have witnessed a slow turning of the tide with some charities and organisations now being run (or partly run) *by* disabled people as opposed to *for* disabled people with more factual and accurate portrayals of disabled people being used both for the purpose of advertising and raising awareness of impairment and disability.

However, some women were fearful that recent and ongoing cuts to local authority budgets and funding to charities and voluntary organisations which have been vital in enabling them to provide fundamental services no longer provided by the statutory sector may result in charitable organisations having to close and their valuable work will cease to exist. Likewise, regular donors to a charity/charities of their choice in difficult economic times may find themselves facing personal financial difficulties and so unable to maintain their regular payments to their chosen charity/charities, thus reducing the charities' sources of income further. In such circumstances some women were concerned that charities would resort to the use of ever more tragic and heart pulling tales in order to maintain levels of donations and in so doing would be reversing efforts in recent times to move away from such modes of fundraising.

Whilst not denying that there would always be scenarios where an individual's circumstances may be considered 'tragic', for example, a suddenly acquired illness or injury that had a massive impact on a person's life and the people closest to them, pitiful representations of physical impairment were widely felt to provide unrealistic and unhelpful reflections of how the majority of disabled women live their daily lives. Similarly, whilst not denying the challenges that living with an impairment may potentially bring to a person's life (particularly when of a life limiting or progressive nature) there was consensus that these were not akin to how disability and impairment were commonly represented across different media forms. Further, by continuing to portray physical impairment in a predominantly negative light, women felt the media would continue to be perceived by disabled people as contributing little of benefit to their overall lives. Therefore, the importance of the UK's media in its many different and rapidly changing technological forms potentially massive role in increasing awareness, knowledge and understanding of impairment and disability within society was strongly emphasised. By true diversity being embraced by the media and building on the witnessed improvement of recent years, this arguably would indirectly make a contribution to improving the self-esteem of disabled people and their quality of life overall through enabling a greater sense of integration and equal participation within twenty-first-century society as opposed to the historical tradition of *us* and *them* – able-bodied and disabled as two separates that never met and were treated differently in all aspects of their lives.

Organisational and Practical Changes

In addition to identifying a number of content changes to the training courses or syllabuses of mental health professionals which women considered needed to happen in seeking to provide in future effective and appropriate provision for disabled women (and men) who experience mental distress, a range of practical considerations which women believed, if applied could singularly or collectively enhance an individual's experience(s) of receiving mental health support were suggested.

Accessibility

Firstly, the vitality of all service locations, consulting rooms and waiting areas to be structurally accessible was consistently emphasised alongside a need for accessible toilet facilities and dedicated parking with a preference for ground floor locations voiced by some due to anxieties about exiting buildings in the event of a fire or lifts being out of order on arriving for appointments. Similar concerns were raised by participants within Jack's (2009) study with Jack having further highlighted the duty of service providers under the new Disability Equality Act (2010) to make reasonable adjustments in order to make their services accessible to disabled people. In situations where this was untenable, then providing an outreach service or offering alternative venues could be examples of reasonable adjustment with the essentiality of service providers consulting with clients about reasonable adjustment likewise emphasised. Whilst for example, telephone or online counselling may not be always considered to be ideal, or would be the form of counselling of a client's choice, such forms can potentially widen access to therapy/counselling for those unable to attend face to face sessions by virtue of their impairment and/or physical health (Jack 2009).

Reduced Waiting for Appropriate Support

Further evidenced by the study findings were participants' concerns over the current waiting times to be seen by a counsellor or other mental health professional with short waiting times having been experienced only by a minority of women for whom the acuteness of their mental distress had necessitated the need for a priority mental health assessment by a professional working in acute mental health. Reduced waiting times for an initial assessment of need were repeatedly highlighted as a major change that needed to happen (though it was widely recognised that long waiting times were problematic for many client groups and not only disabled women). A survey carried out by Mind which looked at waiting times to be seen after referral found that of 500 people (able-bodied) from across the UK who were referred for mental health support, one in five had waited over a year to receive treatment whilst only 8 per cent had been given a choice about the type of therapy they would receive and only 13 per cent a choice as to where therapy sessions or appointments would be held (Mind 2011).

Whilst experiencing lengthy waiting times were shown within the study to have affected women's overall confidence in service provision, analysed data demonstrated a belief that greater confidence in service provision generally would exist if referrers (predominantly the GP), at the point of referral were honest about likely waiting times as opposed to being vague, for example, 'it shouldn't be long' or, 'someone will be in touch'. A number of women further considered their GP had been slow to make a referral to counselling or other mental health services resulting in further delays in addressing their mental distress, and which combined with lengthy waiting to have their needs assessed, was considered to have exacerbated their distress and led to raised stress and anxiety levels. Through listening more earnestly to women's perceptions of the anguish they were experiencing, several women believed that referrals may take place sooner than they had to date experienced and further emphasising the advantageous role of service-user involvement within the training courses of mental health and other professionals who within their work role may work closely with disabled people.

The ability to self-refer to counselling services within their respective academic institutions had been welcomed by two women who had subsequently been offered counselling support within three weeks of referral. However, a number of women expressed caution that a self-refer option for mental health services generally may lead to increased referral rates which potentially could increase waiting times as eligible individuals were screened both for appropriateness and whilst those with the greatest need were identified. Furthermore, concern was voiced that a self-referral option would provide no guarantee that those individuals with the greatest need for mental health support or other forms of treatment would be the ones who self-referred as they may not be sufficiently well to recognise their own distress and are therefore unlikely to self-refer (or may not wish to). Conversely, others claimed that women who did self-refer and who were assessed as having mental health needs may not otherwise have come into contact with mental health services having been reluctant to approach their GP or other appropriate professional. Therefore, whilst the data evidence highlighted both the potential advantages and disadvantages of a self-refer option, overall there was agreement that some form of initial screening by a health, or other appropriate professional was required before services could be accessed so as to ensure their availability to those with identified mental health needs. Making mental health services more accessible and effective, and enabling better access with shorter waiting times are outlined as being a priority for NHS England with £400 million being provided between 2011 and 2015 to provide people with better access to psychological therapies (Department of Health 2012).

Long-term Support

Through providing support that was considered to be appropriate to their needs as disabled women, it was considered would improve women's rating of their experiences of receiving mental health support. Whilst not considering themselves to be in need of ongoing support, women living with progressive or unpredictable impairments spoke of the need for counsellors and allied professionals to recognise that the nature of their impairment may create a need for long-term counselling support with a shared belief that short term counselling was typically ineffective in meeting the psychological needs of women (and men) with progressive and often unpredictable conditions. An ability to access barrier free support from a named worker during times of need, for example, when experiencing a decline in their physical abilities and which in turn was affecting their mental well-being, it was believed would provide women with a service more tailored to their needs whilst consistency of worker would provide greater opportunities for forging a good working relationship. Whilst there was acknowledgement that open-ended counselling provision was not how 'the system' worked, the need for a system in which services were moulded to the client's needs as opposed to the client fitting into the confines of what the service offered was consistently asserted.

In considering herself 'lucky' to have received long-term counselling with a named professional, Claire believed this had been key to enabling her to address some of her mental health issues, in particular her eating distress:

> I knew when I started the counselling that mentally and emotionally I had so much going on and given that previous counselling I'd had ... you blinked and your sessions were over ... so I went with quite low expectations thinking there wouldn't be chance to scratch the surface. But I was fortunate as the counsellor's work was partly funded by a charity organisation and so had more flexibility without promising infinite access ... the counselling lasted a year and what I achieved wouldn't have been possible in a few sessions and building a relationship with the counsellor took time too ... I certainly think long-term support where there's a real need and with the same person. If those things could be available to di people with long-term or progressive conditions that may affect you mentally would go a huge way to improving mental health provision in years to come ... it could make a real difference to people's lives.
>
> Claire (aged 39, acquired spinal illness)

Whilst a minority of women had worked with the same counsellor or mental health professional over a fixed period of time, those who had worked with CPNs within community mental health teams recalled on occasions having to adjust to a change of worker who often used different approaches within their work or had a different personality etc., all of which had to be adjusted to, and not always with success. Similarly, feelings of frustration were expressed by a number of women for whom a reoccurrence of their mental distress had resulted in the need for a new referral to be made which led to further waiting in addition to subsequently being allocated to a new worker who knew little of the woman's circumstances. Having worked with mental health professionals over many years, Philippa voiced her frustrations:

> The days seem long gone when you had a named social worker or other professional who was allocated to you indefinitely ... now you can't ring up and talk to someone without lots of questions being asked which are bad enough when mentally you can cope with them but when you aren't well they are just another barrier to getting through to the person or service you want to have contact with ... The emphasis now seems to be short term work or crisis handling ... basically get professionals in, deal with the immediate problem then move on when in reality you still need the help but mental health services seem to have become a sticking plaster culture.
>
> Philippa (age 36, congenital impairment)

Whilst there was group-wide acknowledgement that as a client group disabled women were not unique in wishing for access to a named professional to support them during episodes of experiencing mental distress, there was consensus that long-term access to a named worker for those with specific identified needs was in future key to increased positive reporting of receiving tailored support from a named individual, service or organisation. However, it was recognised that ever-growing demands on mental health services UK-wide would mean that long-term involvement with a professional was unlikely to become a reality unless an individual's circumstances were deemed to be exceptional.

Improvements in Joint Working

To varying degrees women across the age spectrum had been frustrated by the lack of communication and joint working among the diverse health and social care professionals working alongside them but whose roles were often seen to overlap. Based on both individual and collective experiences, women widely believed that service provision could be improved through community or hospital based professionals both communicating with and working alongside one another, as was deemed appropriate or necessary yet maintaining the principles of confidentiality which to all women were of great importance. Women within Marris's study (1996) who shared their experiences of living with long-term conditions expressed frustration at the lack of a holistic approach to working amongst professionals combined with a lukewarm commitment to joint working between relevant professionals and group-wide women believed that efforts to improve both aspects of working would result in women's physical impairment and mental distress ceasing to be starkly compartmentalised.

As previously discussed, two women with sudden onset acquired impairments were critical of rehabilitation programmes which had focused almost entirely on improving mobility and regaining maximum independence as was deemed possible whilst the psychological impact of acquiring an impairment had been largely ignored. Through integrating a level of psychological support into the rehabilitation programmes of women (and men) with acquired impairments and improved joint working between ward-based health professionals and hospital-based mental health professionals women believed would result in professionals working with a more holistic approach and that the physical and psychological effects of acquiring a sudden onset impairment would cease to be treated in isolation. That the concerns of participants within Morris's study (2004) were mirrored in research several years later (Smith 2010) is disappointing and arguably provides an indicator of the lack of progress made within the areas highlighted. Katy's experiences of the early 1980s were seen to resemble those of women who were receiving support from the same professional groups two decades later:

> I had a social worker who was dealing with the care side of things, an Occupational Therapist who was dealing with the aids etc., district nurses who dealt with the nursing care and then there was the CPN. Well they all came in and filled their various forms which meant me repeating the same stuff the only

> difference was the forms were a different colour yet none of them communicated with each other, there was no joined up thinking ... you just felt like a person who was split up into parts and nobody saw you as a whole person ... some days you could scream. Not long back my care package was reassessed and if I'm honest I was left feeling that things may have changed a bit but a lot of the working practices still seemed to be in the dark ages yet with the technology today I was expecting a lot more.
>
> Katy (age 43, congenital impairment)

Whilst joint working may be hindered by structural and organisational factors, professional perspectives and skills which enable a holistic approach to disability awareness, women believed should be core to the training and education of all health and social care professionals working with the individual and arguably would bring benefit to the individual.

Improved Access to Information

In striving to improve future access to mental health services, a good knowledge of locally-based mental health services that were available for women to access were considered to be vital to ensuring optimum opportunity to access services appropriate to meeting the needs of individuals. Likewise, there was a unanimous belief that easy access to current information about local mental health service availability and their referral processes was vital in enabling appropriate services to be accessed. Furthermore, the need for all information to be jargon-free, to outline clearly what the service or facility provided and its eligibility criteria was highlighted as without this knowledge women could not begin the process of accessing the mental health support or treatment which they had been assessed as requiring or which they considered themselves to require. Participants within Jack's study (2009) further stressed the need for service provision information to indicate clearly that disabled clients are welcomed and to be available in a variety of formats so as to be accessible to those with physical (and sensory/visual impairments) and printed in different languages befitting the local geographical population. Finally emphasised was a requirement for service information to make clear the different therapies and approaches available within any service which would give disabled people the ability to make informed choices about engaging with a process which was considered more likely to empower than oppress.

Several women had received appointments from mental health services which had provided little informative detail, typically highlighted by Philippa:

> I had an appointment letter from a CPN from the local mental health team but it said nothing about what her role was, what the team offered or what I could expect from them ... When she arrived my mum asked for some information about the service but she had nothing and seemed really surprised at being asked. I think services just assume you know what they are about but if you've had no

> previous dealings with them before how can you? She said there may be some stuff online but couldn't really tell us where to look and when we did eventually find something it was more information aimed at professionals working within the service rather than for those using them which wasn't helpful.
>
> Philippa (age 36, congenital impairment)

Helen's experience of gaining knowledge of services which may be beneficial being gleaned from other service-users was shared by a number of women:

> For a while I attended a day care centre for adults with long-term mental health problems and it was through them that I learned about services I could access … that information didn't come from the mental health professionals I was working with yet I saw it as part of their job to let me know about things out in the community which may be helpful. If you don't know these places or services exist how can you start accessing them?
>
> Helen (age 41, congenital impairment)

Women whose impairments affected their ability to easily access public spaces additionaly described the subsequent impact on their ability to access poster or leaflet format information typically located within public buildings such as doctors' surgeries, public libraries or community notice boards. In addition to providing information in traditional paper formats, women applauded service providers who were harnessing recent advances in technology and providing information about mental health services on relevant websites which would assist in ensuring easier access to information about services in particular for individuals for whom leaving their home environment could be problematic. However, caution was called for by women who noted that whilst access to the internet at home is assumed to be becoming the norm, there remain households who choose not to have it, or are unable to meet the costs involved whilst availability should not be assumed to mean ability to make use of it and that therefore provision still needed to be made for accessing information in other formats so as to ensure equality of access for all. A small number of women felt that a perceived reluctance on the part of GPs and mental health professionals to advise women about available services may in part be an attempt to protect services with existing high demands from becoming overloaded whilst cuts to services were resulting in eligibility criteria becoming ever tighter. However, without exception women considered themselves entitled to be fully informed about the availability of mental health services that may be appropriate in meeting their mental health needs.

Provision of Support Groups

Whilst within Chapter 2 it was acknowledged that not all women favoured support groups and preferred instead to confide in close friends, six women considered that in endeavouring to meet their mental health needs a greater availability of support groups for disabled women who were experiencing, or recovering from mental distress would represent a positive development in mental health provision through providing forums where individuals who were experiencing similar difficulties could come together and share experiences. Though factors such as the group's location, the availability of transport and manageable times when groups were held were all recognised as potential barriers to attendance, these women felt that access to a local support group where individuals could spend time in each other's company would be advantageous, in particular whilst waiting to see a counsellor. Additionally, women were seen to have valued other diverse services which some of the groups had offered such as art therapy, relaxation sessions or complementary therapies which had benefited their mental well-being.

Whilst the majority of women expressed a wish to have equal access to the counselling and mental health support services available to able-bodied women given the likelihood of being subject to the same life experiences as able-bodied women, just over half believed that specific support groups for disabled women who were experiencing (or were in recovery from) mental distress had a defined role to play in providing support specifically appropriate to them. Returning home following a stroke (or a period of rehabilitation following a trauma or injury) may be a point of crisis especially when people feel vulnerable and depression can occur. Furthermore, clients who may feel abandoned through a lack of follow-up care may, Herman (1992) believes experience poor self-esteem and despair which potentially may be exacerbated by a lack of emotional support and therefore believes the provision of group support with a shared commonality can be invaluable. However, women considered that such groups would likely only be beneficial if long-term financial support could be guaranteed which in current times was felt unlikely and that closures could impact detrimentally on individuals for whom attending a support group formed an integral part of their support network.

In-patient Care

As the only woman who had experienced in-patient psychiatric care, Claire believed her numerous admissions had enabled her to comprehensively outline the substantial changes which she believed to be necessary if future experiences of in-patient psychiatric care for disabled women were to markedly improve, and with a greater understanding and awareness of disability and impairment among both medical and nursing staff rated as a high priority (Hardcastle, Kennard et al. 2007). Encounters with both nursing and medical staff who assumed Claire's mental distress to be directly linked to her impairment had been commonplace and consequently believing that future experiences of in-patient care would be unlikely to improve until professionals working on acute psychiatric units displayed a shift in attitudes towards physical impairment and were better educated in respect of disability awareness.

Claire's experiences of psychiatric admissions further highlighted the need for ward environments to improve wheelchair access and to cater for the mobility and practical needs of individuals with mobility impairments, for example, the provision of call buzzers, adjustable beds and adapted bathroom facilities which would in turn would likely reduce an enforced dependency on nursing staff for assistance with everyday tasks:

> My last hospital admission, well I was in a bad way yet I knew I didn't want to end up back in hospital because of my previous experiences. In the end it was either go in informally or face the prospect of sectioning. The whole admission just felt undignified and having to ask for help all the while because the ward wasn't easily accessible just made me more miserable and depressed.
>
> Claire (aged 39, acquired spinal illness)

One experience of in-patient care on a specialist psychiatric ward had for Claire represented a positive example of the ways in which mental health services could meet in a holistic and beneficial way the needs of disabled women (and men) who experience mental distress. Located within a specialist hospital, the neuro-psychiatric unit catered for individuals experiencing long-term psychological difficulties or acute mental distress and was managed by nursing staff who, whilst mental health trained also had a wide knowledge base of neurological impairments and the potential ways in which neurological impairments may impact on individual's mental and psychological well-being. Unlike previous admissions to in-patient care which had typically been characterised by days with little structure or sense of purpose, Claire's days on the 10-bed unit were well-structured with a typical day including a counselling session and one to one time with a member of ward staff. Whilst the ward environment was considered to offer a positive example of meeting appropriately the mental health needs of disabled women (and men) who required in-patient neuro-psychiatric care, fellow patients had been frustrated by an average admission waiting time of six months with a two week admission the norm and with little scope for flexibility unless an individual's circumstances were considered by the multi-disciplinary team to be exceptional. The nationwide provision of such specialist units Claire strongly believed would serve to reduce waiting times for admission and would be a welcome future development in providing appropriate mental health provision for individuals with physical impairments who experience mental distress.

Conclusions

Previous chapters have shown how to varying degrees, and for diverse reasons, the majority of women had not considered the mental health support and/or treatment they had received to have sufficiently addressed their mental distress. Within the context of their experiences of working with mental health professionals or mental health organisations, the changes which were considered to be required in providing in future effective mental health services and support for disabled women who experience mental distress have been examined.

From this chapter (and from the study more widely), arguably the strongest message to emerge was for a greater knowledge base of issues relating to disability and impairment to be the foundation upon which mental health and allied professionals can expand their understanding and awareness of issues relevant to the daily lives of people living with a physical impairment. In aiming to provide in years to come mental health services which, UK-wide will meet comprehensively, appropriately and effectively the support needs of disabled people who experience mental distress, such changes were considered to be imperative. Further, a clear need for mental health professionals, through professional training, to become more familiar with the social model of disability and its principles, was felt to be an important way in which individual's awareness and understanding of disability and impairment could be heightened in addition to considering the benefits both for mental health professionals and disabled clients of service-user involvement being routinely included within the training of the practitioners of tomorrow.

Within Chapter 1 it was highlighted how a prolonged inability to access public buildings and spaces was considered to have the potential to impact on mental well-being, with the improvements in structural access which had taken place since the latter decades of the twentieth century having been widely welcomed by all study participants. This chapter has shown the ways in which greater access to the environment had helped to improve women's mental well-being and highlighted the need for mental health professionals to understand and acknowledge the diverse ways in which the removal of structural barriers can and have impacted positively on the physical health and mental well-being of arguably a large majority of the disabled population was strongly asserted. In addition, this chapter has called for professionals working within mental health to gain a greater awareness of how the representation of disability and impairment across different media forms can affect the mental well-being and self-image of disabled women. Historically, disabled people were routinely portrayed as tragic individuals, subjects of pity and sympathy and needing to be cared for. Whilst progress has been made over recent decades in portraying disability more accurately, the vast scope that remains in the early twenty-first century for the media to improve the representation and portrayal of disability, impairment and disabled people in a more accurate and realistic way through its increasingly diverse platforms, was strongly reinforced.

Further highlighted have been a number of practical ways and considerations which it was widely believed would enhance disabled people's future experiences of receiving mental health support; a requirement for service locations within both the statutory and non-statutory sector to meet the access requirements of disabled clients was believed to be vital as were the efforts to be made in reducing waiting times for initial assessments to be undertaken by a counsellor or other professionals. In addition, easier access to and wider availability of service information was rated highly in terms of women being able to begin the process of accessing support.

Through greater efforts being made by mental health and other professionals to communicate with, and work alongside one another it was clearly believed would assist professionals in building a bigger picture of the woman's life which in turn would hopefully result in a greater understanding of the woman's impairment and the ways in which it may impact on different areas of her life. Furthermore, increased joint working in the years ahead it was believed would encourage professionals to shift away from compartmentalising their physical impairment and their experiences of mental distress and in turn would adopt a more holistic approach in which they were seen as a whole person and not as someone defined solely by their impairment.

Chapter 6
Looking to the Future

Introduction

Within the book's introduction, it was highlighted how a key aim of the research undertaken was to produce a study in which the central focus was the experiences of a group of disabled women who had experienced diagnosed mental distress, from their personal perspectives. It further noted how, through the latter decades of the twentieth century a growing body of mental health literature increasingly paid attention to recognising and meeting the support needs of different client groups (women and men) who experienced mental ill-health whilst a likewise expanding disability studies literature paid attention to the differing and specific needs of people living with a physical impairment.

However, by comparison little consideration was given to the support needs of women (or men) who 'fell' into both categories (women living with physical impairments who experienced mental distress) either by writers within the disability studies field or physical impairment or mental health organisations or service providers. Therefore, one of the study's aims, and subsequently this book has been to make a small but hopefully valuable contribution in beginning to fill that gap whilst having also provided the opportunity for a small group of disabled women to talk about their experiences of mental distress, of working with mental health professionals and related topic areas. In so doing, the study sought to answer one overarching question: do UK mental health services in the early twenty-first century currently respond appropriately to the support needs of women with physical impairments who experience mental distress?

In bringing together the dominant messages to emerge from the different topic areas and themes examined within the individual chapters, this final chapter will discuss the potential outcomes both for mental health professionals and the disabled women (and men) with whom they work, if the changes which were highlighted within the research as needing to happen were to became a reality in the years ahead. Simultaneously, the chapter will consider how an increased awareness of the intersections between physical impairment and mental health may transform service provision with consideration for how an alternative approach to gender, disability and impairment would potentially affect the everyday lives of women with physical impairments who experience mental distress.

Physical Impairment: An Inevitability of Mental Distress?

Within Chapter 1 some of the literature and studies which in the latter decades of the twentieth century had examined the subject area of physical impairment and mental health, and subsequently had assumed a causal link between living with a physical impairment and experiencing mental distress were examined. Whilst half of the sample group were seen to have agreed to some degree with a causal link, such a premise was firmly rejected by six women for whom an assumed causal link was believed to be both over-simplified and generalised. Where an experience(s) of mental distress had been considered to varying degrees to be inevitable, any experiences were believed likely to have depended on a variety of factors such as the nature of the individual's impairment (for example, whether acquired or congenital), with the study evidencing a broadly shared view that women with acquired impairments were more likely than women born with their impairments to experience mental distress. Having previously lived with an able-bodied status, women who acquired their impairments had been considered more likely to have an awareness of the historical attitudes towards physical impairment which had prevailed within UK society for much of the twentieth century, whilst the impact of a woman's impairment on her ability to perform everyday tasks independently and the impairment's effect on daily life were also considered to be relevant factors.

However, also evidenced by women's accounts was how those with acquired impairments had strongly considered their experiences of distress to have been associated with what their impairment represented within the context of their lives, for example, possible loss of employment or a relationship breakdown and that their distress had not been linked solely to the impairment per se. For women whose acquired impairments were of a progressive nature, episodes of mental distress had not been experienced as 'a one off'; living with impairments which typically were characterised by fluctuating levels of physical ability, pain and or fatigue had resulted in recurrent episodes of mental distress which women described as having been linked to changes in their physical condition and the subsequent impact of any changes in functional abilities on daily life.

However, the six women living with congenital impairments, (in particular those typically non-progressive in nature, for example, cerebral palsy or spina bifida), did not consider themselves to be exempt from experiencing mental distress with each having recalled in similar terms their first experiences of mental distress as being linked to a realisation of their impairment being a permanent fixture in their lives. Women with congenital impairments (and those with acquired impairments) had also attributed experiences of mental distress to factors such as family bereavement or the loss of significant loved ones or relationship difficulties and highlighted how, as disabled women they could be subject to the same range of life experiences as able-bodied women and these experiences could potentially affect their mental well-being in much the same way as it would affect that of able-bodied women.

Therefore, whilst their individual impairments had been identified by some women as a contributory factor to the onset of their mental distress, group-wide, the absolute need for mental health and allied professionals who may be involved in supporting disabled women who are experiencing mental distress to give greater consideration to a spectrum of factors that may potentially contribute to any experience of mental distress was repeatedly asserted. Likewise, the importance of professionals working with disabled clients to recognise that an individual's experience of living with their impairment will be unique to them, whilst simultaneously acknowledging their individuality, was believed to be imperative.

Further, repeatedly evidenced by the study data was how contacts with mental health professionals (such as community psychiatric nurses, registered mental nurses, clinical psychologists) had, for most women been characterised by individuals who perceived their impairment to be a negative attribute of their life, and viewed by some professionals as a 'tragedy' regardless of whether the woman's impairment had been acquired or been present from birth. Feelings of being pitied and/or patronised by counsellors or allied professionals were likewise widely viewed across the sample group as having stemmed from a professionals overall lack of knowledge, understanding and/or awareness around impairment and disability per se and related issues.

Through mental health professionals displaying attention to the changes which women identified as needing to happen, women firmly believed could lead to positive and advancing steps in the provision of appropriate mental health service provision. Likewise, in the years ahead, through the dedicated commitment of professionals working within mental health to meet effectively and efficiently any individual needs of disabled women (and men) who are identified as being in need of, or are seeking support for, mental distress, women believed and hoped that UK-wide, appropriate mental health services could be provided.

Stigma and Mental Distress

Before revisiting the barriers which many women had experienced in accessing mental health support, within the context of looking at future changes believed to be needed, a short consideration of the issue of stigma may be pertinent. Highlighted within Chapter 4 was how the terminology used by women of different ages when describing their experiences of distress was felt to have been of interest and significance. For example, whilst women aged 50 or over had avoided the use of language such as 'being mentally ill' or 'suffering from mental health problems', such avoidance had been noticeably less evident amongst younger women who spoke more openly about 'being really depressed' or 'feeling anxious and stressed'. Whilst the majority of the women (nine of 12) had considered there to remain a level of stigma attached to people receiving treatment for mental health difficulties, as opposed to a more open acceptance of treatment for physical ill-health, the sense of stigma was felt to have lessened in recent years and was continuing to do so albeit slowly. However, unanimously women considered there to remain significant scope for an improvement of both understanding and awareness of mental ill-health among society alongside a wider recognition of its often indiscriminate nature.

As discussed in Chapter 5, recent years have seen several government campaigns, organised in conjunction with mental health organisations and charities which have aimed both to improve awareness of mental ill-health and to reduce the stigma historically associated with suffering from mental illness whilst simultaneously endeavouring to promote an increased understanding of mental ill-health across society. Additionally, in aiming to both inform audiences and to educate and eradicate within society negative stereotypes of individuals who experience mental distress, a presence on television schedules of programmes featuring storylines involving mental health conditions or documentaries which have examined mental health conditions or mental illness among different client groups, for example *Bedlam* (Channel 4 2013) and *OCD Ward* (ITV 2013) had been widely welcomed. Furthermore, encouraged by a wider discussion and presence of mental health issues generally within the press and on television, a wish to see yet further coverage within the media of an educative and informative nature which would hopefully encourage and promote a more open discussion within mental health was supported wholeheartedly.

Accessing and Using Mental Health Services

In endeavouring to access mental health support, highlighted within Chapter 2 was how efforts to access community and hospital-based services had been experiences that were fraught with difficulties and bureaucracy. In particular, physical barriers to access had been particularly problematic for women who endeavoured to access support prior to the introduction of the Disability Discrimination Act when service providers had no legal obligation to meet the access or other requirements of disabled people. Lengthy waiting times to access services had additionally been a major concern which had caused frustration and anxiety, and only through service provider managers displaying an earnest commitment to reducing waiting times, in conjunction with information about services being more publicised and widely available, would disabled women begin to have a greater confidence in service provision and subsequently, it was hoped, more positive experiences of using services overall. Furthermore, an increased availability of geographically local support groups that catered for any specific needs that a disabled woman may have, it was further believed would assist in improving disabled women's overall perceptions of a range of services being available which offered a good likelihood of being able to meet their needs. Across the sample group the continually high demands being placed on mental health services and the professionals working within them were not disputed. However, through mental health funding bodies UK-wide committing to employing within mental health services (in particular within the statutory sector) sufficient numbers of employees to meet the levels of demand, that assessments of need for short or long term psychological support could be offered within reasonable timescales. In so doing it was hoped this would reduce, as had been experienced by three women the risk of their mental distress being exacerbated whilst waiting to access support.

Once accessed, mental health support (in particular counselling provision) had for the majority of women been offered over a fixed time period. Whilst a minority of women expressed satisfaction both with the support received and the time frame over which it took place, for the majority, the length of time or number of sessions offered by a service or professional had been considered on one or more occasions to have been insufficient in addressing their mental distress and believed that longer-term involvement with a service or professional would have been beneficial to them. In particular, attention was drawn by women living with progressive or life limiting impairments to how access to a named worker would have been, and would if required in future be welcomed through offering consistency of access to a named worker with whom the woman could build a relationship with. Living with impairments which are typically characterised by unpredictable changes in functional abilities and which for a number of women had resulted in repeated episodes of mental distress, the ability to access a named professional during times of need, women believed, would alter their perceptions of services taking account of their individual needs as opposed to a current perception of a one-size-fits-all approach in which a client's needs are 'fitted into' what a service offers. As a group of disabled women, there existed a shared recognition that other client groups may consider themselves to have a need for long-term support. However, the need for professionals to consider the specific needs of women living with life limiting and/or progressive impairments and of how the ability to access long-term support as and when needed, for example, during episodes of decline in their physical abilities may benefit both their physical and mental well-being.

In wishing to see a shift towards mental health support that was more tailored to a woman's individual needs, comparison was made with a recent and ongoing move towards care packages which meet the specific care or support needs of an individual as opposed to an individual fitting into a services or organisation's parameters. For example, since the mid-1990s, following an assessment of a disabled person's needs the individual has been able if they so choose to receive funding from their local authority through which the disabled person is then able to arrange their own care and support in a way that meets their daily needs and wishes. Currently assessments for personalised budgets are being rolled out across the UK providing opportunities for disabled people to have greater control over the support received, from whom and the ways that work for them rather than the service providers; the effect of which on the daily lives of disabled people is maybe too early to comment upon. Within the study, Helen described how direct payments funding had enabled her to arrange the practical care and support she received but importantly had also provided for her mental health support needs with direct payment funding having enabled access to privately funded counselling support and group-wide women supported whole heartedly assessments which in future considered any psychological or mental health needs for which some form of support may be required alongside any physical care needs or requirements.

A shift towards a holistic assessment of needs further supported calls as discussed within Chapter 5 for better communication amongst health and care professionals working with an individual as was deemed appropriate, based on the belief that this would improve confidence in service provision relating both to mental and physical health needs. In addition, it was further hoped that increased joint working would encourage mental health professionals to work within a more holistic approach than to date women considered, based on their own experiences had been evident and that in so doing a disabled woman's physical impairment and mental distress would cease to be compartmentalised and with an individual viewed as 'a whole being'. However, though keen to express optimism about future changes which women felt had the potential to be advantageous to an individual's mental and physical well-being, a scepticism was voiced by women who had worked previously with mental health professionals who spoke enthusiastically of 'multi-disciplinary working' and 'working holistically' but had witnessed few examples of it becoming reality.

Whilst experiences of working with professionals employed within statutory sector organisations or services had for the majority of women been poor or mediocre, conversely, experiences of using services in the non-statutory sector had been rated more highly and with outcomes which overall were rated as both positive and beneficial. The importance of being able to access services such as the Samaritans was strongly emphasised by women who had experienced acute mental distress in particular during night time hours when statutory sector services were routinely uncontactable except for exceptional circumstances. In particular, the ability to access a telephone-based service had been valued by women whose mobility difficulties made it difficult to leave their home environment or who were unable to access public or privately owned transport. The group-wide positive experiences reported by those who used the Samaritans had also been considered relevant within the context of the ongoing debate within recent years as to whether disabled counsellors (or those with previously lived experience of impairment) are the persons best suited to provide counselling support to disabled people. However, there was also recognition that women who reported positive experiences had no knowledge of whether the call handler was able-bodied or disabled and women who used the Samaritans helpline (with one exception) had chosen not to disclose their impairment, their non-disclosure based on not wanting the call handler to assume a causal link between their living with a physical impairment and experiencing mental distress, as had experienced by a number of women when working previously with counsellors face to face.

Counselling and Women with Physical Impairments

Across the sample group, counselling support had been received by 10 of the 12 women and the preference of the large majority to work in counselling with a female counsellor was shown to have been founded predominantly on a belief that as women they would feel more at ease working with someone of their own gender and particularly so if the issues to be addressed within counselling were gender related. However, consistently evident within women's accounts of experiences was that they had not been offered a choice about the gender of counsellor with choice having only been available to individuals who self-funded private counselling.

Also considered within an examination of women's counselling experiences was the ongoing debate in recent decades as to whether disabled people should work in counselling with a disabled counsellor (or one with lived experience of impairment). Whilst data evidence showed the expressed preferences of six women to work with a disabled counsellor to have been rooted in a belief that disabled counsellors would have a better level of understanding and awareness around disability and impairment than an able-bodied counsellor, as a group women did not favour disabled people only working in counselling with counsellors with lived experience of impairment. To adopt such an approach, it was believed would represent a retrograde step at a point in time when disabled people are steadily becoming more integrated within twenty-first-century society. Further, by disabled clients solely working with disabled counsellors (or counsellors with lived experience of impairment), concern was expressed that this would serve to reassert the assumption of a causal link between living with a physical impairment and experiencing mental distress which was suggested within literature and studies discussed within Chapter 1, and which increasingly over the past decade disabled people and academics within disability studies have sought to shift away from and provide evidence to the contrary.

Therefore, the current need both for meaningful debate to take place and for quality research to be undertaken which whole heartedly ascertains the potential benefits or otherwise of disabled counsellors working with disabled people was asserted group-wide with the need for the disabled person's voice to be clearly heard unanimously emphasised. Only in so doing, I would argue, are reliable viewpoints and perspectives likely to be gathered as to whether such provision would be likely in future to result in increased incidences of positive experiences of working with mental health professionals who, through an understanding and awareness of an individual's needs, have worked with clients to address and/or resolve their mental distress.

Further, highlighted within Chapter 4 was how personal experience of impairment was not considered by some women to be imperative in order for the counselling process to be an effective one. Evidenced by the study data was a shared belief that as no two impairments, or experience of those impairments is ever likely to be identical, that a good counsellor should be able to empathise with another person whatever their concerns or life experiences and regardless of being able-bodied or disabled. Based on their personal experiences of counselling, attributes such as the counsellor's character and/or their willingness to listen to and respect a client's views were all identified as being significant whilst factors such as the counsellor's socio- economic background or personality were likewise perceived as key to providing optimum opportunity for forging a good working relationship which had resulted in the individual's mental distress being addressed to their satisfaction.

Despite the expressed preferences of six women to work with a disabled counsellor, none had had their wishes met and only through increased opportunities being made available for disabled people to train as counsellors would disabled clients whose preference was to work with a disabled counsellor, be able to be offered a choice. Historically, barriers to being accepted onto professional training courses have resulted from an individual's lack of recognised academic qualifications, having attended special schools where routinely opportunities to study for academic qualifications had been limited. However, as increasingly in recent decades pupils with a physical impairment have received mainstream education within mainstream schools, so their opportunities to study for the same qualifications as their able-bodied peers have become available and subsequently the option to proceed to further and/or higher education through which the required qualifications for entry into counselling training are routinely gained. Likewise, through course selectors giving much greater consideration to what a disabled individual could potentially bring to a counselling relationship by virtue of their lived experiences of physical impairment and possibly having also experienced mental distress, as opposed to focusing solely on academic qualifications could further lead to an increased availability of disabled counsellors. However, women considered it vital that disabled individuals were not accepted onto counselling training courses solely for the purpose of working with disabled clients or 'meeting quotas' and reinforced the need for recognition that disabled people will likely wish to become counsellors for the very same reasons as able-bodied people, for example, a wish to work with people who are experiencing psychological/emotional difficulties in their lives and consider themselves to have the necessary skills and qualities that are required to work within that role.

Whilst within an expanding body of UK counselling literature in the latter decades of the twentieth century there was, for many years, little discussion of the topic area of counselling and disabled people, more recently the topic has slowly attracted wider discussion and debate though with a handful of exceptions, little has been written from the viewpoint of disabled clients themselves. Thus, in undertaking my research, it was hoped (and is still hoped) that the door will be further opened to meaningful discussion and debate in respect of counselling provision and disabled people amongst counsellors, mental health professionals and disabled people. In giving a voice, in particular to those who have undergone counselling, I believe can only be advantageous in striving for improved provision in the years ahead for those who require the support of mental health professionals and services and that a failure to do so may likely result in current forms of counselling provision and the approaches used by professionals within their work remaining unchanged for the foreseeable future. Furthermore, the findings of the small number of studies of the past decade in which disabled clients predominantly reported negative experiences of working with able-bodied counsellors or other mental health professionals will likely continue to have little impact on changes to service provision which such studies identified as needing to happen in seeking to provide improved and positive counselling experiences.

In addition, whilst recent years have seen the emergence of counselling approaches which have been suggested may be more suitable for working with disabled people than approaches which have traditionally been utilised, their potential to be divisive has been acknowledged, with questions also raised as to whether yet another way of differentiating between able-bodied and disabled people is either wanted or needed. The use of disability counselling approaches have raised concerns of too great a focus being placed on the 'disabled' aspect of an individual's life and resulting potentially in the issues that are central to the woman's distress (and which are not linked to their impairment) being either ignored or entirely overlooked with the necessity of all mental health professionals treating every disabled client as an individual with needs and circumstances that are unique to them firmly reasserted group-wide.

The Concept of Loss

In relation to loss and as discussed within Chapter 3, data evidence indicated a majority belief that at some stage of living with a physical impairment women would experience 'loss' but with marked evidence of variation both in how the concept of loss was understood and how it was experienced. In particular, study findings evidenced how no woman's experience of loss had matched the expectations of established theories of loss and whilst all six women with acquired impairments believed they had 'accepted' their impairments, as individuals none considered themselves to have gone through specified stages before arriving at that point.

Similarly, women whose impairments were present from birth had considered their impairment to be integral to their identity and broadly shared a view point of not feeling able to miss something which had never been experienced such as walking, running etc. Additionally, whilst medical and psychology literatures have routinely portrayed loss as a 'one off' event, the study demonstrated how 'loss' had been experienced at different stages of women's lives and had occurred for example, in relation to barriers to forming friendships or relationships, getting married or having children, one, or all of which were considered to be 'normal' events which a significant proportion of the female population would likely experience during their lifetime.

In recalling personal experiences of loss, women's responses to their impairment were seen to have resonated with more recent, alternative theories of loss and the ways in which they have proposed that individuals respond, or adjust to, living with their impairment. In particular, the experiences of many women were shown to have correlated with how proponents of the dual stages approach believe that disabled individuals respond to their physical impairment, for example, that rather than going through specified stages of grief, women (and men) living with a physical impairment will typically shift between a loss and restoration orientation and with either one being dominant at any one point in time.

Whilst the literature on loss has to date paid scant attention as to whether experiences of loss differ between people born with their impairments, and those whose impairments are acquired, women had widely believed that loss would be experienced differently for women with congenital impairments as opposed to those with acquired impairments. In addition, a shared agreement that loss would be felt more acutely in instances where onset of impairment had been rapid and where the woman's physical mobility, level of independence and overall lifestyle had potentially been substantially affected had been evident. Also emphasised was that whilst a focus on loss may, in some instances be appropriate when working with disabled women, (for example, when working with women with traumatic sudden onset impairments), the need for mental health and allied professionals to recognise and acknowledge the diverse factors that may contribute to an experience of 'loss' was considered to be of great importance. Across the study group and particularly amongst women with acquired impairments, the appropriateness and effectiveness of the mental health support individuals had received in addressing their mental distress had to varying degrees being affected by a perception of professionals having placed too great a focus on loss. Therefore, in keeping sight of whether a consideration of loss within counselling sessions and within the context of an individual's experience of mental distress may be appropriate or not, in wishing to receive effective and appropriate mental health provision in the years ahead, then women believed its usefulness or otherwise to undoubtedly require further purposeful debate amongst relevant parties.

Future Professional Training

In addition to identifying a range of practical and organisational changes which women had believed if applied would improve both service provision and women's overall experiences of using services, Chapter 5 discussed changes which women believed needed to be made as a matter of priority to the training syllabi of counsellors and other mental health professionals who within their future work, may potentially work with disabled clients. Consistently evident within women's accounts of the working relationships with their allocated worker and highlighted across the chapters had been the urgent requirement for mental health professionals to gain a significantly greater understanding and awareness of disability and impairment per se. Until this happened, women strongly believed that service provision would remain unchanged and consequently would continue to meet inappropriately and/or ineffectively the needs of disabled women (and men) who require, or seek support for mental distress.

The introduction of disability equality training and teaching around the social model of disability and its principles, within the courses syllabuses of mental health professionals (with several women also believing that both elements should be included within the training courses of other professionals who may work with disabled clients within a range of capacities, for example, occupational therapists, mental health support workers), it was firmly believed would lead to an improved understanding and awareness of issues relating to disability and impairment and in turn a wider knowledge base overall. Subsequently, in gaining a wholesome awareness of the social model of disability, the professionals of tomorrow, women widely anticipated would be enabled to provide effective and valued support to disabled clients

In addition, study data further drew attention to a seeming lack of available counsellors who specialise in working with disabled clients which was attributed in part to the historical lack of focus on disability issues within training courses and which, combined with an absence of disabled trainees had resulted in disability not being discussed among course leaders or trainees in the way that issues such as gender and race were. Therefore, an increased focus on disability and impairment women believed may lead to counsellors giving consideration to specialising in working with disabled clients. Further, the inclusion of both elements to course syllabuses it was further hoped could potentially offer all trainees an opportunity to identify and address any personal conscious or unconscious prejudices or discriminatory forms of practice within their own contact work with disabled clients. Until mandatory changes to the UK training courses of counsellors were made so as to include disability equality training and teaching around the social model of disability, women voiced dual concerns that counsellors and other professionals who offered psychological support would continue to work within medically informed approaches which viewed their impairment as a 'tragedy'. In so doing, data findings highlighted women's concerns that professionals could potentially continue to be a part of an individual's problems as opposed to playing a role in working towards a resolution of their mental distress. Similarly, until such changes take place, concern was expressed that whilst a minority of disabled women (and men) may have positive experiences of using mental health services, many will continue to receive support that may at best be of a mediocre quality and as such will likely continue to not address their therapeutic needs, with their views remaining disregarded and their voices left silenced.

Further, there was a shared belief in the potential for a greater understanding and awareness of both disability and impairment to be gained through professionals heeding the personal stories of the very individuals who have lived experience both of impairment and mental distress. In so doing, professionals would be enabled to gain a form of knowledge and awareness which could not be gleaned from lecture note taking or book reading in isolation. Whilst the need for counsellors to learn about counselling theory was not disputed, to deny in forthcoming years the voices of individuals' personal experiences women firmly believed would represent a retrograde step in professional practice and the potential for the benefits to be gained by disabled clients within the context of the mental health support received from professionals group-wide were considered to be significant.

Physical Impairment and Social Disability

In recent decades, through the staged implementation of the Disability Discrimination Act and the gradual dismantling of structural barriers, society now arguably has a steadily improving understanding of the physical access needs of disabled people, for example, people are able to understand the concept of wide doorways and ramps enabling access to buildings for wheelchair users or individuals with mobility impairments. As structural barriers within society are steadily eroded thus resulting in an environment that is more accessible to people with physical impairments (though arguably not universally), it may be reasonable to expect that an increased presence and visibility of disabled people in mainstream society will steadily eradicate further in the years ahead some of the historical negative assumptions and stereotypes around disability which remain in society. However, whilst the DDA has slowly improved access for people with physical impairments in mainstream life, even in the utopian dream of a world free from barriers Reeve (2008) believes that psycho emotional disability would still be present within society because of the longevity of prejudicial attitudes and stereotypes about disability.

However, only in recent years have calls begun to be made, mostly by academic writers within disability studies (for example, Thomas 1999 and Reeve 2008) for a greater understanding of the potential of living with a physical impairment to impact on mental and psychological well-being. Whilst disability studies has arguably been excellent in theorising structural disablism which affects what people with physical impairments *can do*, disabling factors which affect disabled people at the psycho emotional level have long been relegated to the domains of personal trouble and the need to be aware of the concept of psycho-emotional disablism and to understand the implications it has for psychological and emotional well-being are arguably especially important for those working in areas such as clinical psychology and counselling. A failure to do so may result in the continued neglect of a form of social oppression which as evidenced by the study has the potential to have substantial and disabling effects on the everyday lives of many disabled people. Whilst the literature has to date not considered to any significant extent the impact of, for example, the impact of the DDA on the mental well-being of disabled people within the context of psycho-emotional disablism, this was considered within my research, with all participants having commented on the positive and diverse ways in which the DDA had affected their mental well-being. For example, the improvements in access to public transport were described by several women as having resulted in feelings of being 'more included' within society through being able to share the same spaces as able-bodied people and as having affected not just what they could 'do' but who they could 'be'. Whilst discussion of this long unconsidered aspect of disablism may be as great a challenge as that of considering other aspects of disablism which have increasingly been debated in recent years, in working towards continuing improvement of attitudes towards, and a greater understanding and awareness of disability and impairment, I believe it to be an important dialogue that needs now to take place.

Additionally, the need for practitioners to be able to distinguish between understandable reactions to the onset of disablism as opposed to emotions that are connected with issues likely to be amenable to psychological input has been highlighted whilst likewise drawing attention to the need for progress to now be made in forging alliances between those working within the disciplines of physical impairment and mental health. In recalling their personal experiences, women wholeheartedly supported such proposals and having been founded, called for ongoing work to build upon and strengthen those links.

Consideration for Future Research and Practice

Within the literature which in recent decades has considered the topic area of women and disability, anthologies have provided an opportunity for disabled women to talk about different aspects of their daily lives, for example, education, access to employment, access to health and social care services, disability benefits, experiences of discrimination and family and personal relationships. However, such texts have predominantly focused on a set point in time with relatively few comparisons having been made between the experiences of women living through different time spans and within different geographical areas. Working within my recent study (Smith 2010) with a group of women with an age span of five decades and living within different UK regions, this enabled comparisons in experiences to be examined and has therefore hopefully made a small but valuable contribution to the literature whilst simultaneously indicating the importance of a generational or life span in context focus in disability research. Furthermore, within women's accounts of areas of their lives within which difficulties or struggles have regularly been encountered these have broadly fallen until recent years within the boundaries of structural barriers to access and historically negative attitudes within society towards physical impairment. Conversely, whilst within my research physical barriers were identified as having prevented access to public buildings and arenas in particular until the latter years of the twentieth century, its focus was to consider the potential of barriers to access and negative attitudes towards impairment to affect mental and psychological well-being.

For the purpose of the research undertaken, whilst a sample group of 12 women may be considered to be small, it endeavoured to provide an opportunity for both women with congenital impairments and women with acquired impairments to share in detail their experiences of mental distress and of using mental health services. Participants were well spread across an adult age range (18–65) and also comprised women who were mothers or had other care responsibilities and women without dependents. In seeking to identify research participants, earnest efforts were made to recruit disabled women from across the UK and from diverse ethnic backgrounds and cultures. However, whilst three women from black and ethnic minorities initially expressed a keen interest to participate, for health and personal reasons each of these women withdrew shortly before the interview process began and therefore the composition of the sample group worked with was 12 women of British white origin. Therefore, in seeking to engage with the experiences and viewpoints of women from ethnic backgrounds and diverse cultures, future research in this area may benefit from efforts being made to recruit participants within geographical areas with a high concentration of ethnic minorities or from organisations that work closely with women from ethnic communities. Indeed, focused studies involving women from specific ethnic minority communities I believe could be fruitful given the different experiences which the limited research to date has shown can result from specific intersections of disability, gender and ethnicity for different groups of disabled people who have used mental health services. In considering future mental health provision which fully meets the mental health needs of disabled women (both with congenital and acquired impairments) who experience mental distress, then the real necessity of listening to the voices and viewpoints of women from different communities, geographical regions, ethnic backgrounds and cultures as opposed to making assumptions about their needs on their behalf cannot be understated.

Furthermore, whilst this text has been founded upon a study which focused upon the experiences of mental distress of women, research which considers the experiences of men with physical impairments who experience mental distress would be valuable and worthwhile and, as with the experiences of disabled women, is already arguably long overdue. A small number of studies which considered disabled men's experiences of mental distress in the 1980s are now somewhat outdated and in light of the dismantling of many environmental structural barriers and shifts in attitudes towards impairment within society which have since taken place, would likely benefit from being revisited; likewise, for the limited studies which have examined the support needs of people with visual or sensory impairments who experience mental distress.

One of the strongest messages to emerge from the study related to changes that women identified as being needed at a service provider level in seeking to increase the incidence of positive reporting of using mental health services; therefore research that examined professional practice that was deemed to be helpful and enabling would be worthwhile. In addition, whilst literature and studies (including my own) have highlighted possible reasons for relationships between disabled people and mental health professionals 'not working', to examine within future work, in more detail than has this text has permitted, 'what works well', I believe, could in the years ahead bring significant benefit to those requiring the support of professionals working in mental health. In particular, research studies whose findings were utilised to feed back into future professional practice could arguably benefit both client and worker. Evident from women's accounts of their working relationships with mental health professionals was how the smallest of actions had made a marked difference to overall experiences of working with an allocated worker and that being listened to or feeling respected had assisted in improving women's self-image and self-worth. Therefore, through building steadily on research which enables the voice of disabled individuals to be heard and their viewpoints listened to, and which identifies high standards of professional practice, like enabling solutions to environmental and structural barriers, respect, humanity and self-esteem would arguably in years to come be restored to the disabled client that the mental health professional is working with, and with a focus on their human existence as opposed to continuing to live as a person defined by their physical impairment.

References

Anthony, K. and Goss, S. 2003 *Technology in Counselling and Psychotherapy*. Basingstoke. Palgrave Macmillan.

Ashurst, P. 1999 *Understanding Women In Distress*. London. Tavistock.

Barnes, C. 1991 *Disabled People in Britain and Discrimination: A Case for Anti-Discrimination Legislation*. London. British Council of Disabled People.

Barnes, C. 1991 Discrimination, Disabled People and the Media Contact No. 70 Winter 45–8. Available online at: The Disability Archive, Leeds University www.leeds.ac.uk/disabilityarchive. Accessed 16 October 2012.

Barnes, C. 2011 Understanding Disability and the Importance of Design for All. *Journal of Accessibility and Design* 1 (1) 54–79.

Barnes, M., Davis, A. et al. 2002 Women Only and Women Sensitive Mental Health Services: An Expert Paper. Report for The Department of Health.

Basnett, I. 1992 Healthcare Professionals and their Attitudes Towards and Decisions Affecting Disabled People. *Handbook of Disability Studies*, Albrecht, G. (ed.). London. Sage. 450–67.

Beckett, C. and Wrighton, E. 2000 What Matters to Me is Not What You are Talking About: Maintaining the Social Model of Disability in Public and Private Negotiations. *Disability and Society* 15 (7) 991–9.

Begum, N. 1990 A Burden of Gratitude: Women with Disabilities Receiving Personal Care. Presentation Paper University of Warwick, Coventry.

Begum, N. 1995 Doctor, Doctor: Disabled Women's Experiences of General Practitioners. *Encounters with Strangers: Feminism and Disability*, Morris, J. (ed.). London. The Women's Press. 94–106.

Begum, N. 1999 From Pillar to Post. *Disability Now*. Issue November 1999.

Berger, R. 1998 Learning to Cope and Survive with Human Loss. *Social Work Today* 28 April 14–17.

Birmingham City Council 1995 An Exploration into Counselling Services for Black and Ethnic Minority Women with Mental Health Problems. Paper by Birmingham City Council, Women's Unit.

Bonnie, S. 2004 Disabled People, Disability and Sexuality. *Disabling Barriers – Enabling Environments* 2nd Edition, Swain, J., French, S., Barnes, C. and Thomas, C. (eds). London. Sage. 74–89.

Bosnich, S. 1985 Women's Experiences of Spinal Cord Injury. *Pride Against Prejudice*, Morris, J. (ed.). London. The Women's Press.

Boswell, G. and Poland, F. 2003 *Women's Minds: Women's Bodies*. Basingstoke. Palgrave Macmillan.

Brearley, G. and Bochley, P. 1994 *Counselling in Disability and Illness*. London. Mosby Press.
British Association of Counselling and Psychotherapy 1998 A Definition of Counselling. Available online at: www.bacp.co.uk. Accessed 7 May 2013.
Brockington, I. 1998 *Motherhood and Mental Health*. Oxford. Oxford University Press.
Brown, I. and Brown, J. 2003 *Quality of Life and Disability*. London. Jessica Kingsley.
Bryant-Jeffries, R. 2004 *Counselling for Progressive Disability*. Oxford. Radcliffe Medical Press.
Burks, H.M. and Steffre, B. 1979 *Theories of Counselling* 2nd Edition. London. McGraw Hill.
Burstow, B. 1991 *Radical Feminist Therapy*. London. Sage.
Busfield, J. 1992 *Women and Mental Health*. Basingstoke. Macmillan.
Busfield, J. 1996 *Men, Women and Madness: Understanding Gender and Mental Disorder*. Basingstoke. Macmillan.
Cahill, C. and Eggleston, R. 1995 Reconsidering the Stigma of Physical Disability: Wheelchair Use and Public Kindness. *Sociological Quarterly* 36 (4) 681–98.
Campling, J. 1981 *Images of Ourselves: Women with Disabilities Talking*. London. Routledge.
Casemore, R. 2006 *Person Centred Counselling in a Nutshell*. London. Sage.
Chaplin, C. 1989 Counselling and Gender. *Handbook of Counselling in Britain*, Dryden, W. et al. (eds). Tavistock. Routledge. 161–74.
Chaplin, C. 1999 *Feminist Counselling in Action*. London. Sage.
Clarkson, P. 2003 *The Therapeutic Relationship*. London. Whurr Press.
Collier, A. 1999 *Being and Worth*. London. Routledge.
Connor, S. and Wilson, R. 2006 It's Important that they Learn from Us for Mental Health to Progress. *Journal of Mental Health* 15 (4) 461–75.
Corker, M. 1996 *Counselling: The Deaf Challenge*. London. Jessica Kingsley.
Corker, M. 2004 Developing Anti-Discriminatory Counselling Practice. *Anti-Discriminatory Counselling Practice*, Lago, C. and Smith, B. (eds). London. Sage. 33–50.
Craib, I. 1998 *Experiencing Identity*. London. Sage.
Craig, A.R., Hancock, K. et al. 1997 Long Term Psychological Outcomes in Spinal Cord Injured Persons. *Archives of Physical Medicine and Rehabilitation* 78 (14) 33–8.
Crawford, D. and Ostrove, J.M. 2003 Sexuality Issues: Who? No! and How: Representation of Disability and the Personal Relationships of Women with Disabilities. *Women and Therapy* 26 (3) 179–93.
Creek, G., Oliver, M. and Zarb, G. 1987 Personal and Social Implications of Spinal Cord Injury: A Retrospective Study. Thames Polytechnic. London. Available online at: The Disability Archive, Leeds University www.leeds.ac.uk/disabilityarchive. Accessed 15 December 2012.

Crisp, R. 2000 A Qualitative Study of the Perceptions of Individuals with Disabilities Concerning Health and Rehabilitation Professionals. *Disability and Society* 15 (2) 355–67.

Crow, L. 1996 Including All of our Lives: Renewing the Social Model of Disability. *Exploring the Divide*, Barnes, C. and Mercer, G. (eds). Leeds. The Disability Press. 55–72.

Currer, C. 2007 *Loss and Social Work*. London. Sage.

Dallton, P. 1994 *Counselling People with Communication Problems*. London. Sage.

D'Ardenne, P. 1999 *Trans-Cultural Counselling in Action* 2nd Edition. London. Sage.

D'Ardenne, P. 2013 *Counselling in Trans-Cultural Settings*. London. Sage.

Davis, K. 1993 The Crafting of Good Clients. *Disabling Barriers – Enabling Environments* 2nd Edition, Swain, J., French, S. et al. (eds). London. Sage. 203–6.

Day, P. 2005 Access to the Built Environment: Is it Improving? Paper presentation. Leeds University, Department of Social Policy. Available online at: The Disability Archive, Leeds University www.leeds.ac.uk/disabilityarchive. Accessed 1 May 2013.

Dennison, L. and Moss-Morris, R. 2010 Cognitive Behavioural Therapy. What Benefits Can it Offer to People with Multiple Sclerosis? *Expert Review of Neurotherapy* 10 (3) 1383–90.

Department of Health 2001 The Expert Patient: A New Approach to Chronic Disease Management for the 21st century. London. Department of Health. Available online at: DoH Publications www.doh.gov.uk. Accessed 14 December 2013.

Department of Health 2002 Women's Mental Health: Into the Mainstream-Strategic Development of Mental Health Care for Women. London. Department of Health. Available online at: DoH Publications www.doh.gov.uk. Accessed 2 September 2013.

Department of Health 2003 Mainstreaming Gender and Women's Mental Health: Implementation Guidance. London. Department of Health. Available online at: DoH Papers www.doh.gov.uk/guidancenotes. Accessed 17 September 2013.

Department of Health 2012 Caring for our Future: Reforming Care and Support. London. Department of Health. Available online at: DoH White Papers www.doh.gov.uk. Accessed 2 January 2014.

Department of Health 2013 Treating Patients and Service Users with Respect, Dignity and Compassion. London. Department of Health. Available online at: DoH White Papers www.doh.gov.uk. Accessed 2 January 2014.

Disability Discrimination Act 1995 (c.50). London. HMSO.

Disability Now 2005 Sex Survey 2005: A Call for Counselling. *Disability Now* June 2005. London. Available online at: www.disabilitynow.org.uk. Accessed 4 June 2013.

Dobash, R. and Dobash, P. 1992 *Women, Violence and Social Change*. London. Routledge.

Doel, M. and Best, L. 2008 *Social Work: Learning from Service Users*. London. Sage.

Doyal, L. 1998 *Women and Mental Health Services: An Agenda for Change*. Buckingham. Open University Press.

Drewitt, J. 1990 Disabilities Nobody Can See. *Disability Now* November 1990. London. Available online at: Disability Now Archive www.disabilitynow.org.uk/archive. Accessed 15 December 2012.

Dryden, W. and Mytton, J. 1999 *Approaches to Counselling and Psychotherapy*. London. Routledge.

Edwards, C. 2012 The Austerity War and the Impoverishment of Disabled People. Paper for National Council of Disabled People. September. Available online at: www.ncodp.org.uk. Accessed 4 January 2014.

Equality Act 2010 c15. Available online at: www.legislation.gov.uk. Accessed 17 December 2013.

Etherington, K. (ed.) 2002 *Rehabilitation Counselling in Physical and Mental Health*. London. Jessica Kingsley.

Feltham, C. and Dryden, W. 1993 *Dictionary of Counselling*. London. Whurr Press.

Fillingham, J. 2013 Changing Needs and Challenging Perceptions of Disabled People with Acquired Impairments. PhD Thesis. University of Birmingham. Available online at: e-theses repository www.etheses.co.uk. Accessed 14 November 2013.

Finkelstein, V. 1980 Attitudes and Disabled People. *Monograph (World Rehabilitation Fund)*. Available online at: The Disability Archive, Leeds University www.leeds.ac.uk/disabilityarchive. Accessed 12 September 2012.

Finkelstein, V. 1987 Images and Employment of Disabled People in Television. Available online at: The Disability Archive. Leeds University www.leeds.ac.uk/disabilityarchive. Accessed 12 September 2012.

Finkelstein, V. 1996 Towards a Psychology of Disability: Psychological Aspects of Impairment. *Disabling Barriers – Enabling Environments* 1st Edition, Swain, J., French, S. et al. (eds). London. Sage. 212–21.

Finkelstein, V. 2001 The Social Model of Disability Repossessed. Available online at: The Disability Archive. Leeds University www.leeds.ac.uk/disabilityarchive. Accessed 11 September 2012.

French, S. 1994 The Attitudes of Health Professionals Towards Disabled People. *Beyond Disability: Towards an Enabling Society*, Hales, G. (ed.). London. Sage. 74–89.

French, S. 1994 *On Equal Terms: Working with Disabled People*. Oxford. Butterworth Heinemann.

French, S. and Swain, J. 2004 Whose Tragedy: Towards a Personal Non Tragedy View of Disability. Available online at: The Disability Archive. Leeds University www.leeds.ac.uk/disabilityarchive. Accessed 12 September 2012.

French, S. and Swain, J. 2004 Disability and Communication: Listening is Not Enough. *Communication, Relationships and Care: A Reader*. Available online at: The Disability Archive, Leeds University www.leeds.ac.uk/disabilityarchive. Accessed 14 September 2012.

Fuhrer, M.J., Hart, K.A. et al. 1993 Depressive Symptomolgy in Persons with Spinal Cord Injury who Reside in the Community. *Archives of Physical Medicine and Rehabilitation* 74 (7) 255–65.

Gido, R. and Dalley, L. 2008 *Women's Mental Health Issues Across the Criminal Justice System*. London. Pearson Education Press.

Gillon, E. 2007 *Person Centred Counselling Psychology: An Introduction*. London. Sage.

GLAD 2003 Into the Mainstream: Strategic Development of Mental Health Care for Women. Response to Women's Mental Health Needs. Publication of Greater London Association of Disabled People. Available online at: www.glad.org.uk. Accessed 12 April 2013.

Glendinning, C., Halliwell, S. et al. 2000 *Buying Independence: Using Direct Payments to Integrate Health and Social Care Services*. Bristol. Policy Press.

Gooding, C. 1996 *A Guide to the Disability Discrimination Act*. London. Blackstone Press.

Goodley, D. 2010 *An Inter-Disciplinary Investigation* 1st Edition. London. Sage.

Goodley, D. and Lamthom, R. 2006 *Disability and Psychology: Critical Introductions and Reflections*. London. Palgrave.

Government Survey 2011 Attitudes to Mental Illness. Available online at: Mind mental health charity website www.mind.org.uk. Accessed 3 January 2014.

Greeley, E. 1996 *The Unclear Path: Life Beyond Disability*. London. Hodder Stoughton.

Griffiths, P. 2002 Counselling and Rehabilitation: The UK Story. *Rehabilitation Counselling in Physical and Mental Health*, Etherington, K. (ed.). London. Jessica Kingsley. 27–45.

Hardcastle, M., Kennard, D. et al. 2007 *Experiences of Mental Health in Patient Care*. London. Routledge.

Harvey, H.J. 1998 *Perspectives on Loss: A Sourcebook*. London. Taylor Francis.

Harwood, R. 2011 Disability, Reasonable Adjustment and Austerity. Paper to British Universities Association Annual Conference 7–9 July 2011. Available online at: The Disability Archive, Leeds university www.leeds.ac.uk/disabilityarchive. Accessed 4 January 2014.

Herman, J.L. 1992 *Trauma and Recovery*. London. Pandora Press.

Hollis, V., Openshaw, S. and Goble, R. 2002 Conducting Focus Groups: Purposes and Practicalities. *British Journal of Occupational Therapy* 65 (1) 2–8.

Hurst, R. 2000 To Revise or Not to Revise? *Disability and Society* 15 (7) 1083–7.

Hurstfield, J., Meager, N. et al. 2006 Monitoring the Disability Discrimination Act. Available online at: link to www.drc.org.uk. Accessed 2 April 2012.

Imrie, R. 1998 Oppression, Disability and Access in the Built Environment. *The Disability Reader. Social Science Perspectives*, Shakespeare, T. (ed.). London. Cassell. 129–46.

Imrie, R. 2004 From Universal to Inclusive Design in the Built Environment. *Disabling Barriers – Enabling Environments* 2nd Edition, Swain, J., French, S. et al. (eds). London. Sage. 287–96.

Jack, S. 2009 Counselling and the Physically Impaired Client: Hearing the Client Voice. Research project for Masters of Arts degree. York University. Paper copy obtained from author.

Johnson, C. 2011 Disabling Barriers in the Person Centred Counselling Relationship. *Person Centred and Experiential Psychotherapies* 10 (4) 260–73.

Keith, L. 1994 *Mustn't Grumble: Writings by Disabled Women*. London. The Women's Press.

Keith, L. 1996 Encounters with Strangers: The Public's Response to Disabled Women and How this Affects our Sense of Self. *Encounters With Strangers: Feminism and Disability*, Morris, J. (ed.). London. The Women's Press. 91–107.

Kennedy, P. 1999 Commentary. *Journal of Evidence Based Mental Health* 2 (2) 58.

Kennedy, P. 2007 *Psychological Management of Physical Disabilities: A Practitioners Guide*. London. Routledge.

Kohen, D. 2000 *Women and Mental Health*. London. Routledge.

Krause, J.S. and Anson, C. 1997 Adjustment after Spinal Cord Injury; Relationship to Gender and Race. *Rehabilitation Psychology* 42 (7) 31–46.

Lago, C. 2007 Counselling across Difference and Diversity. *The Handbook of Person Centred Counselling and Psychotherapy*, Cooper, M., O'Hara, M. and Wyatt, G. (eds). London. Palgrave Macmillan. 251–65.

Lago, C. and Smith, B. 2004 *Anti-Discriminatory Counselling Practice*. London. Sage.

Larocco, N. 2000 Cognitive and Emotional Disorders. *Multiple Sclerosis; Diagnosis, Medicine Management and Rehabilitation*, Burks, J.S. and Johnson, K.P. (eds). Basingstoke. Palgrave Macmillan. 405–23.

Lawson, A. and Matthews, B. 2005 Dismantling Barriers to Transport by Law; The European Journey. Available online at: The Disability Archive. Leeds University www.leeds.ac.uk/disabilityarchive. Accessed 15 April 2013.

Leger, E., Freeston, M.H. et al. 2000 Anxiety and Physical Limitations: A Complex Relationship. *Encephale* 28 (3) 205–9.

Lenney, M. and Sercombe, H. 2002 Did You See that Guy in the Wheelchair Down the Pub? Interactions Across Difference in a Public Place. *Disability and Society* 17 (1) 5–18.

Lenny, J. 1993 Do Disabled People Need Counselling? *Disabling Barriers – Enabling Environments* 1st Edition, Swain, J., French, S. et al. (eds). London. Sage. 233–40.

Lewis, J. 1999 A Case for Specialist Counselling? *News and Views* (British Association of Counselling) 8 (3) 13–15.

Lockwood, S. 1992 Counselling Young Stroke Survivors During Rehabilitation. *Rehabilitation Counselling in Physical and Mental Health*, Etherington, K. (ed.). London. Jessica Kingsley. 79–96.

Lonsdale, S. 1990 *Women and Disability. The Experience of Physical Disability Among Women*. Basingstoke. Macmillan.
Lustig, D. and Strauser, D. 2007 Causal Relationships between Poverty and Disability. *Rehabilitation Counselling Bulletin* 50 (4) 194–202.
Machin, J. 2013 *Working with Loss and Grief: A New Model for Practitioners*. London. Sage.
McKenzie, A. 1992 Counselling for Disabled People Through Injury. Social Care Research Findings No 19. Joseph Rowntree Foundation. York. Available online at: www.jrf/archive/org.uk. Accessed 4 April 2012.
McLeod, J. 1994 *Women's Experiences of Feminist Therapy and Counselling*. Buckingham. Open University Press.
McLeod, J. 1998 *An Introduction to Counselling* 2nd Edition. Buckingham. Open University Press.
Marks, D. 1999 *Disability: Controversial Debates and Psycho-Social Perspectives*. London. Routledge.
Marris, V. 1996 *Lives Worth Living: Women's Experiences of Chronic Illness*. London. Pandora Press.
Mearns, D. and Thorne, B. 2007 *Person Centred Counselling in Action*. London. Sage.
Miles, A. 1988 *Women and Mental Illness*. Brighton. Wheatsheaf.
Mind 2011 Survey of Waiting Times Across the UK. Available online at: Mind mental health charity website www.mind.org.uk. Accessed 2 February 2014.
Mind 2012 It's Time to Talk: It's Time to Change. In conjunction with Rethink. Campaign to tackle mental health discrimination. Available online at: Mind mental health charity website www.mind.org.uk. Accessed 2 February 2014.
Mind 2014 It's the Little Things. In conjunction with Rethink. Campaign to tackle mental health discrimination www.mind.org.uk. Accessed 2 February 2014.
Moore, M. 2013 User Involvement in Services for Disabled People. *Disabling Barriers – Enabling Environments* 3rd Edition, Swain, J., French, S. et al. (eds). London. Sage. 190–97.
Morgan-Jones, R. 2002 Counselling after Hearing Loss. *Rehabilitation Counselling in Physical and Mental Health*, Etherington, K. (ed.). London. Jessica Kingsley. 109–30.
Morris, J. (ed.) 1989 *Able Lives: Women's Experience of Paralysis*. London. The Women's Press.
Morris, J. 1991 *Pride Against Prejudice: Transforming Attitudes to Disability*. London. The Women's Press.
Morris, J. 1993 Gender and Disability. *Disabling Barriers – Enabling Environments* 1st Edition, Swain, J., Finkelstein, V. et al. (eds). London. Sage. 140–51.
Morris, J. 1998 Feminism, Gender and Disability. Seminar Presentation. February 1998. Available online at: The Disability Archive, Leeds University www.leeds.ac.uk/disabilityarchive. Accessed 4 April 2013.
Morris, J. 2002 People with Physical Impairments and Mental Health Support Needs: A Review of the Literature. Joseph Rowntree Foundation. York. Available online at: www.jrf.org.uk/archive. Paper copy obtained from author.

Morris, J. 2004 One Town for My Body: Another for My Mind: Services for People with Physical Impairments and Mental Health Support Needs. York. Joseph Rowntree Foundation Publications.

Morris, R. 2012 'I am really fearful of what is going to happen to me in the near future' The Impact on Disabled People of Cuts and Changes to Benefits and Services. Dissertation submitted for MA in Disability Studies, Leeds University. Available online at: The Disability Archive, Leeds University www.leeds.ac.uk/disabilityarchive. Accessed 4 January 2014.

Multiple Sclerosis Essentials Information sheet No. 10 2009 Mood, Depression and Emotions. London. Multiple Sclerosis Society.

Multiple Sclerosis Essentials Information sheet No. 21. 2011 Exercise and Physiotherapy. London. Multiple Sclerosis Society.

Nairn, K. and Smith, G. 1986 *Dealing with Depression*. London. The Women's Press.

Nattiello, P. 2001 *A Person Centred Approach: A Passionate Presence*. Ross on Wye. PCCS Books.

Neimeyer, R. and Anderson, A. 2002 Meaning Reconstruction Theory. *Loss and Grief*, Thompson, N. (ed.). Basingstoke. Palgrave Macmillan. 45–65.

Nosek, M. and Hughes, R. 2003 Psycho-Social Issues of Women with Physical Disabilities: The Continuing Gender Debate. *Rehabilitation Counselling Bulletin* 46 (4) 221–4.

Office for Disability Studies 2007 Improving Information on Services to Disabled People. London, ODS. Available online at: The Disability Archive, Leeds University www.leeds.ac.uk/disabilityarchive. Accessed 12 October 2013.

Oliver, J. 1995 Counselling Disabled People: A Counsellor's Perspective. *Disability and Society* 10 (3) 227–43.

Oliver, M. 1987 *Walking Into Darkness: The Experience of Spinal Cord Injury*. Basingstoke. Macmillan.

Oliver, M. 1990 *The Politics of Disablement*. Basingstoke. Macmillan.

Oliver, M 1995 Developing an Understanding of Societal Responses to Long Term Disability. Available online at: The Disability Archive, Leeds University www.leeds.ac.uk/disabilityarchive. Accessed 14 April 2013.

Oliver, M. 1996 *Understanding Disability: From Theory to Practice*. Basingstoke. Macmillan.

Oliver, M. 2004 If I Had a Hammer: The Social Model in Action. *Disabling Barriers – Enabling Environments* 2nd Edition, Swain, J., Finkelstein, V. et al. (eds). London. Sage. 18–31.

Oliver, M. 2004a Disabled People and the Inclusive Society: Or the Times They Really Are Changing. Public Lecture, University of Greenwich. Available online at: The Disability Archive, Leeds University www.leeds.ac.uk/disabilityarchive. Accessed 14 April 2013.

Oliver, M. and Barnes, C. 2010 Disability Studies: Disabled People and the Struggle for Inclusion. *British Journal of The Sociology of Education* 31 (5) 547–60.

Olkin, R. 1999 *What Psychotherapists Should Know About Disability*. New York. The Guildford Press.

Olkin, R. 1999a The Personal, Professional and Political: When Women have Disabilities. *Women and Therapy* 22 (92) 87–104.

Olkin, R. and Pledger, C. 2003 Can Disability Studies and Psychology Join Hands? *American Psychology Journal* 58 (4) 296–304.

Parkinson, G. 2006 Counsellor's Attitudes Towards Disability Equality Training. *British Journal of Guidance and Counselling* 34 (1) 29–34.

Paulson, B., Truscott, D. and Stuart, J. 1999 Clients Perceptions of Helpful Experiences in Counselling. *Journal of Counselling and Psychology* 46 317–24.

Payne, N. 1999 *Loss and Bereavement*. Buckingham. Open University Press.

Pelletier, R.J. 1989 Barriers to the Provision of Mental Health Services to Individuals with Severe Physical Disability. *Journal of Counselling Psychology* 32 (3) 422–30.

Perkins, R. et al. 1997 *Women In Context: Good Practice in Mental Health Services for Women*. London. Good Practices in Mental Health.

Perry, J. 1993 *Counselling for Women*. Buckingham. Open University Press.

Pilgrim, D. 2005 *Key Concepts in Mental Health*. London. Sage.

Prideaux, S. 2006 Good Practice for Providing Reasonable Access to the Built Environment for Disabled People. Available online at: The Disability Archive, Leeds University www.leeds.ac.uk/disabilityarchive. Accessed 15 April 2013.

Priestley, M. 2003 *Disability: A Life Course Approach*. Cambridge. Polity Press.

Prime Ministers Strategy Unit 2005 Improving the Life Chances of Disabled People. London. PMSU. Available online at www.gov.uk. Accessed 4 February 2013.

Pring, J. 2008 More Choice, More Control, More Life. Article Feature, *Disability Now* Issue 4 34–36. Available online at www.disabilitynow.org.uk. Accessed 5 April 2013.

Prior, P. 1999 *Gender and Mental Health*. Basingstoke. Macmillan.

Proctor, G. 2008 Professionalization: A Strategy for Power and Glory. *Therapy Today Journal* 19 (8) 31–4.

Reeve, D. 2000 Oppression within the Counselling Room. *Disability and Society* 15 (4) 669–82.

Reeve, D. 2002 Negotiating Psycho-Emotional Dimensions of Disability and their Influences on Identity Constructions. *Disability and Society* 17 (5) 493–502.

Reeve, D. 2003 Encounters with Strangers: Psycho-Emotional Dimensions of Disability in Everyday Life. Paper presented for Disability Studies Conference. Lancaster University. Available online at: Lancaster University www.cedr.co.uk. Accessed 4 April 2013.

Reeve, D. 2004 Psycho-Emotional Dimensions of Disability within Relationships between Professionals and Disabled People. Paper presentation. Department of Applied Social Studies. Lancaster University. Available online at: Lancaster University www.cedr/co.uk. Accessed 4 April 2013.

Reeve, D. 2005 Towards a Psychology of Disability: The Emotional Effects of Living in a Disabling Society. *Disability and Psychology: Critical Introductions and Reflections*, Goodley, D. and Lawthom, R. (eds). London. Palgrave. Chapter 7.

Reeve, D. 2008 Psycho-Emotional Disablism: A Neglected Dimension of Disability? Keynote Paper. Cornwall Disability Research Network. November 2008. Available online at: Lancaster University Disability Studies Conference website www.cedr.ac.uk/archive. Accessed 4 April 2013.

Reeve, D. 2008a Negotiating Disability in Everyday Life: The Experience of Psycho-Emotional Disablism. PhD Thesis. University of Lancaster. E-copy provided by author.

Reeve, D. 2012 Psycho-Emotional Disablism: The Missing Link. *Handbook of Disability Studies*, Watson, N., Roulstone, A. and Thomas, C. (eds). London. Routledge. 78–92.

Reeve, D. 2013 Counselling and Disabled People: Help or Hindrance? *Disabling Barriers – Enabling Environments* 3rd Edition, Swain, J., French, S. et al. (eds). London. Sage. 255–62.

Reeve, D. 2013a Psycho-Emotional Disablism and Internalised Oppression. *Disabling Bariers: Enabling Environments* 3rd Edition, Swain, J., French, S. et al. (eds). London. Sage. 92–9.

Robinson, C., Martin, J. et al. 2007 Attitudes Towards and Perceptions of Disabled People: Findings from a Module of 2005 British Attitudes Survey. Prepared for Disability Rights Commission. Available online at: The Disability Archive, Leeds University www.leeds.ac.uk/disabilityarchive. Accessed 7 March 2013.

Robinson, C. and Stalker, K. 1998 *Growing Up with a Disability*. London. Jessica Kingsley.

Rock, P.J. 1996 Eugenics and Euthanasia: A Cause for Concern for Disabled People, Particularly Disabled Women. *Disability and Society* 11 (1) 121–7.

Sadovnik, A.D., Remick, R.A. et al. 1996. Depression and Multiple Sclerosis. *Journal of Neurology* 46 626–32.

Samaritans and McNamara, J. 2000 Present Dangers: The Impact of Physical Impairment upon Mental Well-Being. Research Project carried out by The Samaritans. London.

Sancho, J. 2003 Disabling Prejudice: Attitudes to Disability and its Portrayal on Television. Report of research undertaken by the British Broadcasting Commission, the Broadcasting Corporation and the Independent Television Commission. Available online at: The Disability Archive, Leeds University www.leeds.ac.uk/disabilityarchive. Accessed 15 December 2012.

Sapey, B. 2002 Impairment, Disability and Loss: Reassessing the Rejection of Loss. *Illness Journal of Crisis and Loss* 12 (1) 90–107.

Sapey, B. 2004 Disability: What Loss and Whose Loss? Seminar paper, Leeds University, April 2004. Available online at: Lancaster University. Centre for Disability Studies www.cedr.co.uk. Accessed 12 December 2012.

Sapey, B., Stewart, J. and Donaldson, G. 1996 The Social Implications of Increases in Wheelchair Use. Department of Social Studies. Lancaster University. Report 2004. Available online at: The Disability Archive, Leeds University www.leeds.ac.uk/disabilityarchive. Accessed 15 December 2012.

Scope 2013 Have the Paralympics Improved the Daily Lives of Disabled People? Report by Scope. Available online at: Scope website www.scope.org.uk. Accessed 5 January 2014.

Scope 2014 End the awkward. Scope Campaign in Working Towards Improving Attitudes Towards Disabled People and Ending Awkwardness. Available at Scope website www.scope.org.uk. Accessed 6 May 2014.

Segal, J. 1989 Counselling People with Disabilities and Chronic Illnesses. *Handbook of Counselling in Britain*, Dryden, W. and Woolfe, R. (eds). Tavistock, Routledge. 65–79.

Segal, J. 2002 Counselling People with Multiple Sclerosis in Rehabilitation Counselling. *Physical and Mental Health*, Etherington, K. (eds). London. Jessica Kingsley. 47–62.

Shah, S. and Priestley, M. 2011 *Disability and Social Change: Private Lives and Public Spaces*. Bristol. Polity Press.

Shakespeare, T. 1994 Cultural Representations of Disabled People: Dustbins for Disavowal. *Disability and Society* 9 (3) 293–306.

Shakespeare, T. 2000 Disabled Sexuality: Towards Rights and Recognitions. *Disability and Society* 18 (3) 159–66.

Shakespeare, T. 2006 *Disability Rights and Wrongs*. London. Routledge.

Shakespeare, T. and Watson, N. 2001 The Social Model of Disability: An Outdated Ideology. *Research in Social Sciences and Disability* 2 9–21.

Sheldon, A. 2001. Disabled People and Communication Systems in the 21st Century. PhD Thesis. University of Leeds. Available online at: The Disability Archive, Leeds University www.leeds.ac.uk/disabilityarchive. Accessed 15 January 2013.

Sheldon, A. 2013 Women and Disability. *Disabling Barriers – Enabling Environments* 3rd Edition, Swain, J., French, S. et al. (eds). London. Sage. 70–77.

Siegert, R.J. and Abernethy, D. 2005 Depression in Multiple Sclerosis: A Review. *Journal of Neurology, Neurosurgery and Psychiatry* 76 469–75.

Smart, J. and Smart, D. 2006 Models of Disability: Implications for the Counselling Profession. *Journal of Counselling and Development* 84 29–44.

Smith, G. and Cox, D. 1999 *Women and Self Harm*. London. Routledge.

Smith, J. 2003 Access To, and the Provision of Mental Health Support Services for Women with Physical Impairments. Dissertation for MA in Disability Studies, Leeds University. Available online at: The Disability Archive, Leeds University www.leeds.ac.uk/disabilityarchive.

Smith, J. 2005 Women with Physical Impairments, the Experience of Loss and the Role of Social Factors on Mental Health and Well Being: A Critical Review of the Literature. Dissertation for Masters Degree in Social Research. University of Birmingham.

Smith, J. 2010 Women with Physical Impairments and Mental Distress. PhD Thesis. University of Birmingham. Available online at: www.ethesesbham.co.uk.

Social Policy Research Unit 1992 The Availability of Counselling for Disabled People: A Review Commissioned by the Joseph Rowntree Foundation. University of York. Available online at: www.jrf.org.uk/archive. Accessed 11 May 2012.

Spinal Cord Injury Association 2005 Emotional Support and Spinal Cord Injury. Available online at: www.spinalinjury-net. Accessed 16 July 2012.

Stainton, T. and Boyce, S. 2004 I Have My Life Back: Users Experiences of Direct Payments. *Disability and Society* 19 (5) 444–54.

Stenager, E.N., Jensen, K. et al. 1992 Suicide and Multiple Sclerosis: An Epidemiological Investigation. *Journal of Neurological Neurosurgery and Psychiatry* 55 542–5.

The Stroke Association 2006 Improving the Life Chances of Disabled People. Available online at: The Stroke Association website www.stroke.org.uk. Accessed 2 November 2012.

The Stroke Association 2012 Psychological Effects of a Stroke. The Stroke Association Factsheet. Available online at: Stroke Association Website www.stroke.org.uk. Accessed 3 May 2013.

The Stroke Association 2013 Feeling Overwhelmed. Report by the Stroke Association on the psychological effects of stroke. May 2013. Available online at: The Stroke Association website www.stroke.org.uk. Accessed 6 September 2013.

Swain, J. and French, S. 2000 Towards an Affirmative Model of Disability. *Disability and Society* 15 (4) 669–82.

Swain, J., French. S., Finkelstein, V. and Thomas, C. (eds) 2004 *Disabling Barriers – Enabling Environments* 2nd Edition. London. Sage.

Swain, J., Griffiths, C. and Heyman, B. 2003 Towards a Social Model Approach to Counselling Disabled Clients. *Journal of Guidance and Counselling* 31 (1) 65–74.

Syder, D. 1998 *Wanting to Talk: Counselling Case Studies in Communication Disorders*. London. Whurr Publishers.

Tew, J. 2011 *Social Approaches to Mental Distress*. Basingstoke. Palgrave Macmillan.

Thomas, C. 1998 Parents and Family: Disabled Women's Stories about their Childhood Experiences. *Growing Up with a Disability*, Robinson, C. and Stalker, K. (eds). London. Jessica Kingsley. 85–96.

Thomas, C. 1999 *Female Forms: Experiencing and Understanding Disability*. Buckingham. Open University Press.

Thomas, C. 2001 Medicine, Gender and Disability: Disabled Women's Healthcare Encounters. *Healthcare for Women International Journal* 23 245–62.

Thomas, C. 2004 Developing the Social Relational in the Social Model of Disability: A Theoretical Agenda. *Implementing the Social Model of Disability*, Barnes, C. and Mercer, G. (eds). The Disability Press. Leeds. 32–47.

Thomas, C. 2007 Sociologies of Disability: Contested Ideas. *Disability Studies: A Medical Sociology*. Palgrave Macmillan. Basingstoke.

Thomas, C. 2007 The Disabled Body. *Real Bodies*, Evans, M. and Lee, E. (eds). Basingstoke. Palgrave. 64–79.

Thomas, P., Gradwell, L. and Markham, N. 2004 Defining Impairment within the Social Model of Disability. Paper presentation. Available online at The Disability Archive, Leeds University www.leeds.ac.uk/disabilityarchive. Accessed 5 July 2013.

Thompson, N. (ed.) 2002 *Loss and Grief*. Basingstoke. Palgrave.

Tighe, C.A. 2001 Working at Disability: A Qualitative Study of the Meaning of Health and Disability for Women with Physical Impairments. *Disability and Society* 16 (4) 511–29.

Titchkosky, T. 2001 *Reading and Writing Disability Differently: The Textured Life of Embodiment*. Toronto. University of Toronto Press.

Triskel, N., Jade, R., Weston, H. and Patterson, W. 2007 Making Therapy Accessible to Disabled People. British Association of Counselling and Psychotherapy: Information Sheet G11. Lutterworth Press.

Turner, R.J. and Noh, S. 1988 Physical Disability and Depression: A Longitudinal Analysis. *Journal of Health and Social Behaviour* 29 (12) 23–7.

UPIAS 1976 *Fundamental Principles of Disability*. Union of the Physically Impaired Against Segregation.

Ussher, J. 1991 *Women's Madness: Misogyny or Mental Illness?* London. Wheatsheaf Publishers.

Vasey, S. 1992 A Personal Experience of Living with a Physical Impairment. *Mustn't Grumble: Writings by Disabled Women*, Keith, L. (ed.). 1994. London. The Women's Press. 66–74.

Vernon, A. and Qureshi, H. 2000 Community Care and Independence; Self Sufficiency or Empowerment? *Critical Social Policy* 20 (2) 25–7.

Walker, M. 1992 Women in Therapy and Counselling. Buckingham. Open University Press.

Watermeyer, B. 2009 Claiming Loss in Disability. *Disability and Society* 24 (1) 91–102.

Wates, M. 1994 Self-Respect. *Mustn't Grumble: Writings by Disabled Women*, Keith, L. (ed.). London. The Women's Press. 75–87.

Webb, S.B. 1993 Disability Counselling: Grieving the Loss. *Counselling Approaches in the Field of Disability*, Robertson, S. and Brown, R. (eds). London. Chapman and Hall. 102–20.

Webbe, L. 2010 Facing out the Elephant. Feature Article. *Disability Now* Summer 2010. Available online at: Disability Now website www.disabilitynow.org.uk. Accessed 8 April 2013.

Wilson, S. 2003 *Disability, Counselling and Psychotherapy: Challenges and Opportunities*. London. Palgrave Macmillan.

Wimpenny, P. and Costello, J. 2011 *Grief, Loss and Bereavement: Evidence and Practice for Health and Social Care Practitioners*. Routledge. London.

Withers, S. 1996 The Experience of Counselling. *Beyond Disability: Towards an Enabling Society*, Hales, G. (ed.). London. Sage. 64–79.

Woodin, S. 2006 Social Relationships and Disabled People: The Impact of Direct Payments. PhD Thesis. University of Leeds. Available online at: The Disability Archive, Leeds University www.leeds.ac.uk/disabilityarchive. Accessed 5 February 2014.

Woolley, M. 1993 Acquired Hearing Loss: Acquired Oppression. *Disabling Barriers – Enabling Environments* 1st Edition, Swain, J., French, S. et al. (eds). London. Sage. 78–82.

Zarb, G. 1995 *Removing Disability Barriers*. London. Policy Studies Institute.

Zarb, G. and Oliver, M. 1987 Ageing with a Disability. Available online at: The Disability Archive. Leeds University www.leeds.ac.uk/disabilityarchive. Accessed 6 September 2012.

Index